Community, Physicians, and Inequality

Community, Physicians, and Inequality

A Sociological Study of the Maldistribution of Physicians

William A. Rushing

Vanderbilt University

Lexington Books

D.C. Heath and Company
Lexington, Massachusetts
Toronto   London

Library of Congress Cataloging in Publication Data

Rushing, William A.
    Community, physicians, and inequality.

    Includes index.
        1. Physicans–United States–Supply and demand.
    2. Medicine–Specialities and specialists–United States.
    3. Community health services–United States–Location.
    4. Community organization. I. Title. [DNLM: 1. Physicians–Supply
    and distribution–United States.   2. Social planning–United States.
    W76 R953c]
    RA410.7.R87   331.1'26   73-20925
    ISBN 0-669-91686-2

Published simultaneously in Canada

Printed in the United States of America

International Standard Book Number: 0-669-91686-2

Library of Congress Catalog Card Number: 73-20925

For my parents

Contents

List of Figures

List of Tables

Preface

This book began in 1969 when I was head of Sociological Studies in the Tennessee Mid-South Regional Medical Program (TMS/RMP), holding a joint appointment with that agency and the Department of Sociology, Vanderbilt University. As a new member of TMS/RMP I was particularly impressed by the plight of many rural and economically depressed communities in the region. Citizens of these communities stated that there was a shortage of physicians in their communities, and they argued that TMS/RMP was not doing very much to help, and indeed, that it was actually helping communities where physician manpower was already high more than it was helping them—the wealthier communities were getting most of TMS/RMP project funds.

On the basis of data provided by TMS/RMP and some that was available in public documents I investigated the situation and found that the concerns were well founded. I then developed a conceptual framework in which it was possible to understand why physicians and TMS/RMP resources were so unevenly distributed in the communities of the region. Part of the result of that effort was published in 1971 in *Social Problems* under the title, "Government Policy, Community Constraints, and the Distribution of Medical Resources." The general thesis was that since the allocation of TMS/RMP funds was dependent on a grant mechanism, it gave an advantage to communities where physicians were in high supply, and that community differences in the supply of physicians stemmed from general social, economic, and demographic differences between communities. The effectiveness of TMS/RMP in responding to the communities most in need was constrained by community conditions over which it had no control.

During 1970 and 1971, I explored the relationship of these same conditions to physician manpower for all counties in the United States, drawing on data from the 1960 United States Census and the county location of all United States physicians in 1966 as published by the American Medical Association (AMA). Although the results were in many respects similar to those for the Tennessee Mid-South Region, they indicated that the conceptual framework was inadequate both with respect to some of the statements it contained as well as things that it omitted. The framework presented in Chapter 3 and the general outline of Chapter 16 of the present book began to take shape.

In 1974, the American Association of Medical Colleges made available to me certain data from their Longitudinal Study of physicians who entered medical school in 1956. These data included physicians' places of practice in

1972, career plans during the senior year, and several background characteristics, including places of birth. The analysis of these data permitted me to round out and complement the analysis based on the relationships between county characteristics and physician ratios. Findings for the AAMC study identified somewhat more specifically some of the conditions and processes that contribute to the uneven distribution of physicians. They also allowed the identification of some of the effects of suburbanization on the distribution of physicians, which was not possible with the data derived from documents published by the AMA and U.S. Bureau of the Census. With the addition of these findings the book began to take its current form.

The book represents an effort to understand an important social problem using the conceptual knowledge and methodological skills of a sociologist. Although it does, I think, contribute a little to our understanding of American communities and American society, it is more properly considered a form of "applied" sociological research than "pure" research. The central effort is directed to understanding a concrete problem of society rather than understanding the nature of society itself.

Consequently, the book is addressed to formulators of public policy and members of the medical community as well as social scientists. Effort therefore has been made to eliminate as much jargon as possible and to present the results in such a way that they are readily understood by those not versed in technical statistical analysis. To this end, the result of several regression analyzes have been presented in graphic form. Although regression lines add nothing to the technical analysis, they do provide visual presentations that may aid those who are unfamiliar with the meaning of such things as regression and correlation coefficients. In spite of these efforts, I suspect too many readers will consider that I have fallen short of my goal.

A note of gratitude is in order for a number of individuals and agencies, without whose assistance the book would either not have been written or would have taken even much longer to complete. The response of Paul M. Teschan and Robert Metcalfe, formerly Director and Associate Director of the Tennessee Mid-South Regional Medical Program, to an early paper out of which this book grew were helpful, as were the assistance of Charles Geiger, Charles Johnson, Ruth Hagstrom, Yaw Chin Ho, and George E. Trent, also former members of TMS/RMP, in providing needed data and technical assistance.

Computer assistance was provided by a number of individuals, and include George Wade, W. Jeff Reynolds, and especially Ned Becker, all from Vanderbilt University. They along with a number of other graduate students (Jack Esco, John Ehnes, Neil Fleming, Thomas James, Paul Placek, Erica Powell, Susan Smith, George Wade, and Frank Wier) also provided me with a forum to discuss many aspects of the book; I thank them for their patience in listening to what I had to say, and for their ideas.

A special thanks goes to the American Association of Medical Colleges for providing important data from the AAMC Longitudinal Study. Ayres D'Costa and Rosemary Yancik, Principal Investigator and Project Director of the Study, and Sherman Williams and Jerry Weston of the National Center of Health Services Research, made it possible for me to obtain these data.

A number of people read the entire manuscript and their comments were always helpful, even if their suggestions were not always followed. They include Stan Czamanski of Cornell University, Glenn Fuguitt of the University of Wisconsin, Lewis Lefkowitz of Vanderbilt University, David L. Miles of the University of Alabama, Kay D. Rushing, Nashville, Walter S. Slocum of Washington State University, and Mayer N. Zald of Vanderbilt University. Discussions of portions of this book with Ivar Berg and James Blumstein of Vanderbilt University and Michael Zubkoff of Dartmouth College were helpful. Valuable advice was obtained from Bradley Hertel, Tony Oberschall, and Frank Wier, all of Vandervilt University, concerning some of the technical details of statistical analysis. Special gratitude goes to Cindy Miller, who typed the manuscript (parts of it several times), compiled tables, and constructed charts and graphs.

As in so many work activities, writing a book sometimes intrudes into one's life so much he does not spend as much time with his family as he would like, or should. Writing this book was no exception. Many hours were spent at the typewriter, in the library, and studying data which would have otherwise been spent more enjoyably with Claudia, Kay, and Todd. Without their understanding, patience, and support, this book would have been far less pleasant to write and my loss in not spending more time with them would have been even greater.

Community, Physicians, and Inequality

1 Introduction: The Medical Crisis and Physician Manpower

This book is about an important American social problem—the shortage of physicians in many communities in the United States. The problem is frequently referred to as the "maldistribution" of physicians, that is, the wide discrepancies between communities in physician manpower. For example, in 1971 according to the American Medical Association (Roback 1972) there were 143 active non-federal physicians per 100,000 population for the nation as a whole,[a] but in this same year there were 133 counties that had no physician and many others that had less than 50 per 100,000 population. Whereas some communities have far more than their proportionate share of physicians, other communities have far less—hence the claim that physicians are maldistributed.

No one argues that all areas and communities should have the same number of physicians per unit of population; probably everyone recognizes that a completely even distribution of physicians is not desirable (Fahs and Peterson 1968), although no one has established the amount of inequality that *would* be acceptable. Most agree with the economists Henry B. Steele and Guston V. Rimlinger that "the spatial distribution of physicians in relation to population [is] highly uneven in the United States [and] must be considered less than ideal . . . ." (Steele and Rimlinger 1965, p. 182). The existence of such wide discrepancies, with physician manpower that is higher than any industrial society in the world,[b] leaves many persons perplexed.

Several explanations have been offered for the condition, most of which focus on some characteristic of the field of medicine itself. Some emphasize characteristics of *individual physicians*; the problem is said to be due to the economic motivation of physicians that leads them to concentrate in high income communities and to neglect communities where incomes are low. Other explanations focus on actions by the *professional association* of physicians, such as the American Medical Association's attempt to limit the number of physicians so that we are said to have an overall shortage of physicians—in spite of the fact that we now have more physicians per unit of population than most societies of the world. Still other explanations emphasize the *institution of medical care*—to its

---

[a]Population figures for computing the U.S. ratio are based on the estimate of Sales Management, Inc., which is reported in G.A. Roback (1972).

[b]By way of comparison, England and Wales have 111 and 83 per 100,000 population.

1

"nonsystem" character and the absence of systematic planning among physicians as well as among other health professions and agencies involved in the delivery of health care.

Although factors from all three levels—individual, associational, and institutional—are no doubt involved in the problem, the thesis of this book is that an important cause of the problem is found at a more general level—the structure of *society* and of *general* social and economic differences between *communities*. The problem is too complex to be attributed to the actions of physicians alone (e.g., to their economic behavior and their efforts to limit the supply of physicians). It is part of a more general pattern of social and economic differences between communities, and physicians have had little to do with creating these general differences. Moreover, rather than being a nonsystem when viewed in relation to the social and economic differences between communities, the medical institution—at least in reference to the distribution of physicians—manifests a most orderly and systematic character. The maldistribution of physicians is only one part of a broader macrosocioeconomic pattern that has a predictable and discernible system character to it. It is rooted in the structure of American society and in the general differences between communities within American society.

The thesis of the book is stated in general terms by Robert N. Nisbet and Roland L. Warren. Nisbet states that "to uncover the causes of [a social] problem, [we must identify its] determining context." The "determining context" may include many things that are "accepted by society as unobjectionable, even good" (Nisbet 1971 pp. 19, 9). But regardless of the valuation of the context as good or bad, it is in terms of *it* that the problem is examined. Specifically, community differences in physician manpower must be viewed from the perspective of the community contexts in which those differences exist. In general terms, Warren states, "a closer look at some of the underlying processes taking place within the community may afford a backdrop against which the community conditions which we interpret as 'problems' can be understood as part and parcel of the system of community living which has developed in America. The alternative approach is to take each problem out of its situational context and treat it in isolation from the basic community conditions which produced it" (Warren 1972, p. 15). This suggests that the maldistribution of physicians should be viewed as interrelated with other aspects of communities, and as a symptom of underlying causal processes that have their origins in the general character of communities. It is viewed this way in this book.

This is not to say that aspects of the field of medicine are not important. But all operate within a more general context. The institutional characteristics of medicine, such as physician specialization and physician dependence on hospital facilities, are particularly important; but they do not operate in isolation from the broader context of society and community, and their influence on the distribution of physicians is shaped in important ways by this broader context.

Institutional characteristics of medicine and the structure of communities interact. Specifically, the influence of specialization and hospital facilities on the distribution of physicians varies, depending on the community context.

The approach of the book, therefore, is sociological. It views physician manpower as a community property and as related to other community properties. Explanation for the maldistribution of physicians is sought primarily in communities, social institutions, and the interaction between the two, not in the characteristics of individuals. The approach would seem to be self-evident. It is in terms of differences between communities, after all, that the problem exists; consequently, it is in terms of general differences between communities that an explanation of the problem is sought.

The book is also concerned with social policy. A basic thesis, derived from the theoretical framework and the empirical analysis that is guided by that framework, is that major changes in the distribution of physician services will not come about until policies that are designed to redistribute medical services recognize that a major locus of the problem is in general differences between communities and not solely in the attitudes, motives, values, and other personal characteristics of individual physicians. A more equitable distribution of medical services will more likely come from a change in intercommunity relationships and the intercommunity organization of medical services than it will from efforts either to increase the supply of physicians or to change the motives, attitudes, or other characteristics of physicians.

The Problem in Broader Perspective: The Paradox of American Medicine

The distributional problem is only one aspect of the so-called medical crisis. In several ways American medicine is a paradox. We now spend almost 8 percent of our gross national product on medical care and this is more than double the percentage we spent 40 years ago; scientific and technological developments have made it possible to treat many crippling and life-taking diseases successfully; many millions of dollars have been spent since World War II in building hospital facilities, so that today all but a relatively small proportion of the population reside in close proximity to a hospital; and the supply of physicians per unit of population is at least as high as it was 30 to 40 years ago. In spite of all this, much dissatisfaction is expressed about medical care in the United States.

The criticisms are several. One is economic. The proportion of the gross national product (GNP) devoted to medical care shows a steady rise in recent years—5.9 percent in 1964, 6.5 percent in 1967, 7.1 percent in 1970, and 7.6 percent in 1972 (Rice and Cooper 1973); at this rate it will be near 10 percent by 1980. The cost of medical care, therefore, has increased to the point where it creates financial hardships for many individuals and families. Also, many persons are now questioning the medical profession's long-standing claim that Americans receive the best medical care in the world. Indeed, some contend that the quality of medical care in the United States is too poor and point to the unfavorable comparison between the United States and other nations in infant mortality and overall death rates (infant mortality is generally accepted as the most sensitive single index of the health status of an entire population; such statistics show that from 11 to 17 countries have lower rates than we do [cf. Rutstein 1967, pp. 11-28]).

Another issue relates to access to medical care. In spite of the comparatively high physician-to-population ratio, there is much talk about a doctor shortage, which some contend is due to the policy of the American Medical Association to restrict the number of medical-school graduates (Kessel 1970). Also, in spite of increases over the years in the removal of financial barriers to medical care through medicare, medicaid, and increased coverage by private insurance carriers, charges are made that large segments of the population (e.g., blacks, low income groups, rural communities) do not receive medical care that is equal to that received by other segments. And still others claim that medical practice has become so scientific-technical that physicians may have forgotten the "human dimension" and emotional aspects that have been traditionally associated with the practice of medicine (Fields 1970).

It is not surprising, therefore, that on the basis of its assessment of American health care, the President's National Advisory Commission on Health Manpower concluded that "there *is* a crisis in American health care" (National Advisory Commission on Health Manpower, Vol. 1 1967, p. 2; emphasis in original). And the general public, and to a somewhat lesser degree physicians themselves, seems to agree. In 1971 a total of 61 percent of a representative sample of the American public agreed that "there is a general 'health crisis' in the U.S. that will require some basic changes in how medical services are made available," and among physicians 64 percent either agreed that we are "in the midst of a major national health crisis" or that there are "serious problems" in medicine (but no crisis) (Strickland 1972, pp. 32-43).

The idea of a medical crisis has not gone unchallenged. And the challenge comes not only from members of the American Medical Association, either. For example, Harry Schwartz, a member of the editorial board of the *New York Times*, makes a "case for American medicine" (1972). He argues that the quality of medical care in the United States is not inferior to other affluent nations, and contends that most middle-age Americans recognize that American medicine today is superior to what it was in previous years. He believes, as do others, that the health of the nation will improve and the death rate will drop primarily as the result of such things as cleaner air, gun control, lower alcohol usage, lower drug and fat consumption, and safer driving. He is less persuasive concerning the issue of costs, although some do contend that it is no worse to spend 10 percent of the GNP on medical care than it is to spend this much, and more, on other things.

There is little room for disagreement on the maldistribution issue, however. Physicians from low manpower communities view the matter with alarm (Parker and Tuxhill 1967, p. 322), and supporters of American physicians, such as Schwartz and the American Medical Association, admit to the existence of the problem (Schwartz, 1972, pp. 70-77, 90; American Medical Association, 1973; see also Bible 1970, p. 11.). A number of documentaries by the mass media as well as research studies have been directed to it. More than a few claim that it constitutes one of the most important and persistent problems in medical care today (cf. Marshall et al. 1971, p. 1556). And certainly, the existence of over 100 American counties with no physicians and many others where physician manpower is in short supply are matters beyond dispute. The problem has not been created by political rhetoric, and it does not exist as a mental image in the minds of some people with no factual basis in the world. The problem is real.[c]

Aspects of the Problem

The first thing that usually comes to mind when one thinks about communities that have a shortage of physicians is that medical care is limited or non-existent to members of the communities in question. Still, the relevance of physician manpower statistics for gauging the availability of health services is sometimes questioned; for example, some claim that many persons in communities with low physician manpower go outside the community for medical care. Rashi Fein observes, however, that there are "geographic limits beyond which available services cannot usually be 'exported' or dispensed. As a result, the quantity of physicians' services available in a geographic area is directly related to the number of physicians available in and around that area" (Fein 1967, p. 72), and Bond Bible contends that "the maldistribution of physicians in certain areas [deprives] communities of immediate access to medical care" (Bible 1970, p. 11). Indeed, evidence does indicate that areas in which physician manpower is in short supply tend also to be areas in which per capita physician contacts are fewer and the average time per contact is shorter than in areas where manpower is not so limited (Rimlinger and Steele 1963, p. 9). Evidence also suggests that physicians in physician shortage areas work longer hours than physicians in other areas, and as a consequence they are characterized as being overworked (cf. Bible 1970; Crawford and McCormack 1971; Fein 1967; Parker and Tuxhill 1967; and Rimlinger and Steele 1963). Thus, not only is the uneven distribution of physicians a fact beyond dispute, but inequities in medical care and work pressure on physicians appear to be consequences of this fact.

---

[c]For an opposite view see George Melloan (1973), who asserts that the problems of health care in the United States have gotten their crisis status largely because Senator Edward Kennedy labeled health care a "crisis" in 1971.

Although heightened public awareness of this condition seems to have emerged only in recent years, the problem itself is not new. Nor is its recognition entirely new. In 1942 and 1945 Joseph W. Mountin, the then assistant surgeon general of the United States, and his associates published a series of papers dealing with the distribution of physicians in the United States between 1923 and 1938. They reported wide disparities between regions, states, and counties in the number of physicians per 100,000 population (Mountin, Pennell, and Nicolay 1942a, 1942b, 1942c, and Mountin, Pennell, and Brockett 1945). A number of recommendations have also been made since then and some have been implemented in an effort to improve the situation. Authors have recommended the establishment of hospital facilities in communities with low physician manpower as a means by which communities could attract physicians (cf. Mountin, Pennell, and Brockett 1945, p. 184, and Williams and Uzzell 1960). Additional medical schools have been advocated; and according to some the "national concern over deficits in and maldistribution of medical manpower" has been an important factor in the development of many medical schools since World War II (Marshall et al. 1971, p. 1556). Numerous communities have provided free clinics and other inducements in order to attract more physicians.

Yet, after the establishment of hundreds of hospital facilities and thousands of hospital beds in communities short on physician manpower, the addition of over 30 new medical schools since 1945, and the offer by communities of rent-free clinics and other advantages to physicians, community inequities in physician manpower continue to exist. For example, the Sears-Roebuck Foundation has attempted to attract physicians to small and usually rural areas by helping communities build clinics. It is reported that 162 were built between 1956 and 1971, but by July 1971, 52 had been vacated or had been converted to other uses (Star 1971, p. 16). Many individual stories have been told of communities that built hospital and other medical facilities to attract and keep physicians only to find that they were unable to attract physicians or even to keep those physicians they had. This suggests that the roots of the condition do indeed extend beyond the field of medicine and into the broader society.

More recent programs to deal with the problem have been advocated, and some have been established. The Comprehensive Health Manpower Training Act of 1971, the National Health Service Corp, and former President Nixon's proposal to provide initial funding for eight new medical schools strategically located in the United States represent attempts to cope with the problem. The use of paramedical or allied health personnel in place of physicians in physician shortage communities has been recommended (e.g., Fein 1967; Marshall et al. 1971, p. 1563; and Sadler, Sadler, and Bliss 1972). The recruitment of students from rural economically depressed communities to medical schools has been proposed in hope that they will return to their home communities, on the ground that physicians currently practicing in such communities tend to have been reared in those communities (cf. Bible 1970; Hassinger 1963; and Parker and Tuxhill 1967).

Greater "outreach" responsibility by medical schools, in the form of continuing education and residency-internship programs for communities short on physicians has been proposed. Some of these programs are too new to permit an assessment of their impact, and in any case few systematic efforts have been made to examine their effects. Several will be examined in this book.

Approach of the Book

Studies of the geographical distribution of physicians have shown that a number of variables are related to the distribution of physician manpower. (For a recent listing of variables, see James Cooper, Karan Heald and Michael Samuels 1972). These include various economic indices (per capita income, economic growth rate), size of the population, level of urbanization, physician income, cultural and recreational resources, educational level of population, age and racial composition of the population, physician background (e.g., rural versus urban), physician specialization, and location of medical schools. In an effort to bring some understanding to this array of relationships, the question may be asked as to the relative importance of the different variables. If some (ideally one) are found to be very important and the rest are of minor importance, the latter may be ignored and attention focused on the former. This may lead to greater understanding of the major underlying causes of the maldistribution and this in turn to the development of policy programs that deal effectively with the problem.

In approaching the problem this way, the research strategy is to examine the relationships of many variables to physician manpower in some form of multivariate statistical model. The relationship between the several variables and the supply of physicians (usually the number of physicians per 100,000 population) is examined to see to what extent combinations of these variables are able to predict physician manpower better than one variable alone, or to determine which among the several variables is the best predictor of physician manpower. In such studies the following kind of question is asked: "Given the units of analysis under consideration [metropolitan areas], what single predictor variable will give us a maximum improvement in our ability to predict values of the dependent variable [the number of physicians per 100,000 population]" (Joroff and Navorro 1971, p. 431).

The approach offers an important advantage. It permits the handling of a number of variables simultaneously and thus the identification of what may be the most important ones. There are limitations to the approach, however, and its use may lead to questionable results. This could occur if the many predictor variables are themselves highly correlated. Then statistically controlling for variable (Z) while examining the statistical effect of (X) on (Y) may in effect also control for (X). In this case the partial correlations may be difficult to interpret. Also, a measure of the combined effects of all such variables (multiple correlation) does not consider that some of the independent variables may be causally related and that these relationships are themselves part of a causal chain in which physician manpower is involved. Moreover, the approach in itself does not distinguish between different types of variables. For example, community wealth, level of urbanization, physician specialization, and number of community hospital facilities may all be correlated with the number of physicians per 100,000 community population. However, the first two are clearly of a different order from the latter two. Community wealth and urbanization are more general characteristics of communities than the mix of physician specialties and number of hospital facilities in a community. Their influence on the community is far more general than the number of physician specialties and hospital facilities, which are largely confined to the medical sector. Community wealth and urbanization constitute conditions or contexts for physician specialists and hospital facilities, but the number of physician specialists and hospital facilities never constitute a context for community wealth and urbanization. Moreover, community wealth and urbanization may exert significant effects on the relationship between the mix of physician specialities and hospital facilities in the community, but the mix of physician specialities and hospital facilities are of much less significance for the relationship between community wealth and urbanization.

In sum, statistical techniques in themselves do not provide a guide for selecting variables to study, which relationships among the various variables are important to examine, or the types of distinctions to make between different variables. Decisions concerning these matters must be made within some theoretical framework. These decisions are not always made in ways in which the investigator may wish. Variables may have to be selected because of the availability of data rather than because of their theoretical importance. Frequently, one may have to compromise since variables obviously cannot be measured unless appropriate data are available. Much of the analysis in this book is also based on data available in published sources. As a result, measures of some of the variables fall short of the theoretical ideal and only approximate the theoretical properties of the variables in question. Nevertheless, the approach in this book differs from other studies in the theoretical perspective that guides the selection of variables for study and the analysis and interpretation of relationships between those variables. Although the study includes many of the variables that have been investigated by others, they are selected for study because they are considered to be causally related to the distribution of physicians on theoretical grounds. The major variables include community wealth, the percentage of residents living in urban areas, community population size, community background of physicians, physician specialty, and community hospital facilities. Theoretical distinctions are made between these variables.

One distinction is between community characteristics and individual physician characteristics. For example, community wealth and percentage of urban residents are community characteristics whereas community background of physicians and physician specialty are individual characteristics. (As will be seen, however, the latter two characteristics may be aggregated to compose community characteristics. For example, community backgrounds of physicians may be aggregated to form an index of community production of physicians, and physicians may be aggregated by specialty to produce an index of community manpower for different specialty groups.) Individual characteristics and their effect on the maldistribution of physicians are examined within the broader context of community characteristics. For example, the effect of the tendency for physicians to practice in communities similar to those in which they were reared is viewed in terms of institutional differences between communities which in turn result in certain types of communities producing, as well as recruiting, a disproportionate number of physicians.

In addition, a distinction is made between different community characteristics. A distinction is drawn between *general* characteristics of community and *medically specific* characteristics. As noted above, community wealth and urbanization are considered general characteristics, whereas hospital facilities and the number of physician specialists relative to the number of general practitioners are community characteristics that are specific to the medical sector. The former constitute a context for the latter. Also, community wealth and urbanization are considered as contextual variables for community population size. Specifically, the effect of community size on the distribution of physicians is seen to vary depending on community wealth and urbanization.

Part I, Chapters 2 through 6, describes the relationships between the general characteristics and the physician ratio for counties and smaller communities within counties. Chapter 2 examines the relationship between the county physician ratio and county wealth and percentage of county residents living in urban areas. Two general patterns in this relationship are observed. One pattern is the continuation of a long historical trend, whereas the other appears to have emerged in more recent years. Chapter 3 presents a general theoretical statement that provides a causal explanation for the results in Chapter 2. The next three chapters investigate several implications of that framework. Chapter 4 studies county differences in the production of physicians and the relationship between the income and urban levels of physicians' counties of origin and counties of practice, and both are seen as contributing to the maldistribution of physicians. County differences in socialization institutions are viewed as the cause of differential production rates, as well as a major factor in the nature of the relationship between income and urban levels of physicians' counties of origin and counties of practice. Chapter 5 extends this analysis by examining the consequences this relationship has for counties of different income and urban levels. Chapter 6 examines the relationship of size of place to physician manpower.

The relationship is viewed in terms of the suburbanization process, which in turn is viewed in relationship to the theoretical framework presented in Chapter 3.

The major aim of these chapters, then, is to show that difference in physician manpower is only one aspect of more general community differences. Communities are viewed in terms of three general factors: the economic sector, the size-density of the population (percentage of residents living in urban areas), and the service-occupational sector. The three are considered as interdependent and related to processes that extend beyond the boundaries of the community. Since physician manpower is part of the service-occupational sector, community physician manpower is viewed in terms of its relationship to the community income base and size-density of the population. Physician manpower, then, is considered as another social and economic resource of the community and subject to the same causal factors as other community social and economic resources.

Part II, Chapters 7 through 11, examines the effects of two medically specific characteristics on the distribution of physicians within the framework of the general patterns and theoretical interpretations presented in Chapters 2 through 6. Chapters 7, 8, and 9 show that the processes identified earlier effect the distributional patterns of different types of physicians in different ways. Chapter 7 shows the different distributional patterns for different types of physicians, Chapter 8 differences in the relationship between income and urban levels of counties of origin and counties of practice, and Chapter 9 the differential effect of suburbanization. The central thesis of these three chapters is that specialization within medicine interacts with more general social and economic patterns in its effect on the maldistribution of physicians. The relationship between hospital facilities in counties and county physician manpower is explained in Chapters 10 and 11. Chapter 10 observes that such a relationship exists only for specialists and that the relationship even here varies depending on community wealth and urbanization and probably suburbanization. Then in Chapter 11 the relationships between hospitals, specialists, and generalists are viewed from the perspective of functional alternatives, which states that there may be no inherent one to one correspondence between the institutions of a community and the functions performed by the institutions. Particular institutions are not necessarily indispensable for society; the same function may be performed by different institutions (Merton 1957, pp. 32-37). With the historical increase in hospitals and decrease in general practitioners, it is argued that hospitals have become functional alternatives to general practitioners for some of the functions that modern specialty medical practice makes necessary. The possible changing role of hospitals in medical care is thus examined within the context of the relationship between generalists and specialists. Therefore, in Chapter 11, I move from a *distributional* perspective to an *organizational* perspective. The increase in specialization is viewed in terms of increased structural differentiation within medicine, and referral patterns are viewed as integrative mechanisms. Hospitals then are viewed as emerging substitutes or functional alternatives for generalists in the referral process to specialists. The implications of these patterns for the distribution of physicians are developed.

Part III, Chapters 12 through 16, examines several alternative policies and their effects (potential or actual) on the distribution of physicians. Chapter 12 examines the probable effects of programs designed to change characteristics of physicians, specifically, programs designed to create more general and family practitioners and a higher proportion of physicians who were reared in rural and low-income areas. Chapter 13 considers the potential effects of an increase in the supply of physicians and an equalization of the demand for medical services through some form of universal health insurance. In Chapter 14, policies of locating more medical training institutions in areas of physician shortage are examined. Then in Chapter 15, the effects of two programs that are oriented toward making changes at the community level—Hill Burton Construction Program and Division of Regional Medical Program Service—are investigated. All programs in Chapters 12 through 15 are examined in light of the constraints of nonmedical characteristics of communities. In Chapter 16 an alternative plan is outlined and is examined in light of the results and perspective presented in Chapters 2 through 15.

A Note on the Data

Data for the study are from several sources. Most data on the practice locations of physicians are an American Medical Association publication, which gives the counties of practice for almost all U.S. physicians as of 1966, and the American Association of Medical College Longitudinal Study, which gives the physicians' place of practice in 1972 for a sample of physicians who entered medical school in 1956 and who graduated in 1960. Most data on the characteristics of physicians' places of practice are from a variety of publications by the U.S. Bureau of the Census. The AMA data on physicians for 1966 form the basis for part of the analysis in Chapters 2, 7, and 11, and all of the analysis in Chapter 10, while data from the AAMC Longitudinal Study form the basis for part of chapters 2 and 7 and most or all of the analysis in Chapters 4, 6, 8, 9, 10, and 12.

The use of data for 1966 requires a comment. At the time when the analysis of physicians for all U.S. counties was conducted, the latest year on which data were available for social and economic characteristics for all U.S. counties was 1960; consequently, data on physicians for a year close to 1960 was desirable. Data for 1966 were chosen because the AMA publication for this year contained a more complete set of data on the number of physicians and other medically relevant characteristics by county than publications for previous years. The use of data for a later date would not have represented any particular advantage.

First, AAMC data for physicians' places of practice in 1972 are used to supplement AMA data for 1966. Also, comparison of the distribution of all physicians for 1966 with those in the AAMC Study for 1972 allows the identification of recent changes in the distribution of physicians that might not have been as noticeable if a later year than 1966 had been chosen. In addition, the primary objective of the data analysis is to identify patterns of relationships between the distribution of physicians by place of practice and the social and economic characteristics of places. Although there may have been some small changes overall in the proportional distribution of physicians in U.S. communities since 1966, such changes have undoubtedly been small and would have little if any effect on the pattern of relationships observed for physicians as of 1966.

Conclusion

In contrast to the view adopted by many persons, in this book the medical institution, and specifically the distribution of physicians across American communities, is considered a part of an overall system or scheme of things. To argue that the medical institution is a "nonsystem" is to contend that there are no systematic relationships between it and other aspects of society. The argument also implies that the problems (as well as positive aspects) of American medicine are the results of the particular motives and values of physicians. This views the problem too atomistically, and asserts moreover that there is no apparent coherence or order in the behavior of physicians. The assumption of this book is different. Physicians' behavior, like the behavior of any occupational group, is patterned and is part of broader sets of events. And it is in terms of such broader patterns that the distribution of physicians in communities in the United States is to be understood.

Part I

General Patterns

2 Community Wealth, Urbanization, and Physician Manpower

Most of the concern about the shortage of physicians has focused on low income and rural areas. This is reflected in the congressional statement on "National Health Priorities" in the National Health Planning and Resources Development Act of 1974. The Act states that congress finds that "primary care services for medically underserved populations, especially those which are located in rural or economically depressed areas" deserve "priority consideration in the formulation of national health planning goals." The concern is also reflected in a number of studies that have discovered an inverse relationship between the physician manpower of geographic areas and the per capita income and percentage of residents within the area who live in urban areas. The areas that have been the object of study, or the units of analysis, have been regions, states, selected counties and towns within states and regions, and Standard Metropolitan Areas (Benham, Maurizi, and Reder 1968; Cooper, Heald, and Samuels 1972; Fahs and Peterson 1968; Fein 1967; Fein and Weber 1971; Held 1973; Joroff and Navorro 1971; Marden 1966; Parker, Rix, and Tuxhill 1969; Rimlinger and Steele 1963; and Steele and Rimlinger 1965). A limitation of these studies is that there may be wide variation within the areas studied with respect to income and urbanization levels; this is especially true when the areas are regions and states. It is conceivable, therefore, that in many instances the local communities with the most physician manpower may not be the wealthiest or most urbanized within the area. In instances where the analysis is based on smaller units, such as towns and counties (Fahs and Peterson 1968; Parker, Rix, and Tuxhill 1969), analysis is limited to only a small proportion of all such units in the United States and their representativeness is unknown.[a] Consequently, analysis based on smaller units that are known to be representative of the entire country is needed.

This chapter presents the results of an investigation of the relationship between physician manpower and the income and urban levels for all counties in the United States. It also presents the results for the distribution of a sample of physicians who entered medical school in one year (1960). On the basis of these results two general types of explanations are discussed. One focuses on the reasons physicians have for locating in some areas rather than others, in which case the cause of maldistribution of physicians is viewed in terms of the

---

[a]An exception is the study of counties in the twenties and thirties by Mountin and associates (1942a, 1942b, 1942c, and 1945).

motives of physicians. This approach will be examined in light of the results of the chapter, and one of its major limitations will be noted. The other explanation locates the cause of the maldistribution in factors external to physicians. A framework for viewing the findings of this chapter from this perspective will be presented in the next chapter.

There are several reasons for limiting the analysis in this chapter to the roles of economic and urban factors. One reason is to provide a descriptive picture of the maldistribution. The chapter will thus provide an assessment of the general belief that physicians are in short supply in rural and low income communities. Also, income and urbanization are the two major aspects of communities within which the effects of other variables take place; consequently, the effects of these two variables need to be examined before additional variables are included in the analysis. In addition, both in frameworks that focus on individual motivation and in the one presented in the next chapter, county income and urbanization (as it is measured in this study) would be expected to be significantly related to county physician manpower. Limitation of the analysis to just these two variables allows the two types of interpretations to be seen in contrast.

Another reason might also be mentioned. Because of the limited resources available for the study, limitations had to be imposed on its scope. Consequently, although data are available for a number of other county characteristics, data for only a few of them were obtained. The criteria used in selecting variables were (1) evidence from other research that indicated the variable was important and (2) whether the variable would be expected to be related to physician manpower on purely theoretical grounds.

The chapter will serve one other purpose. It will introduce the two sets of data on physicians from which much of the analysis in subsequent chapters will be drawn.

All United States Physicians and Counties

In examining physician manpower for a population it is necessary to control or standardize for the total population since the number of physicians (as well as most other occupational groups) will be highly correlated with the total population (cf. Marden 1966). Two procedures are available for doing this. The most common method is to divide the number of physicians in each area by the total population of the area. This gives a physician-to-population ratio for each area, and thus expresses the number of physicians in the area relative to the total population in the area. The ratio is usually multiplied by some constant, usually 100,000, so that the physician manpower for an area is expressed as the number per 100,000 persons. The other method is to use the absolute number of physicians, but when examining the relationship between the number of physicians and other characteristics of the population (e.g., per capita income) the total population is a control variable in a multiple regression equation. Although most studies have used the first procedure, some are based on absolute numbers (Mardin 1966; Reskin and Campbell 1974) and one has used both the absolute number and the ratio (Benham, Maurizi, and Reder 1968). Although there are good reasons for using either method, the more common method is used here. Measures for physician manpower by county are the number of physicians per 100,000 county population. (Methodological problems in using the ratio and the reasons for using it rather than the absolute number are outlined in Appendix A.)

One of the difficulties of investigating physician manpower is that the number of physicians reported for an area (county, state or region) varies depending on the source of the data. It will also vary in the same source for different classifications of physicians—all physicians, federal and nonfederal; all nonfederal active physicians; all nonfederal physicians, including inactive physicians; or all active nonfederal physicians "providing patient care," excluding medical researchers, faculty, and administrators. The analysis in this section is based on the number of active nonfederal physicians classified as primarily engaged in patient care, thus excluding all who are primarily in research, faculty, and administrative positions, but including interns and residents. Since interns and residents are included, the number is inflated to the extent that it is viewed as the number of permanent county physicians who are primarily engaged in patient care. However, the elimination of physician teachers, researchers, and administrators, many of whom perform some direct patient care service, depresses the figure. Since interns-residents and teachers-researchers-administrators are disproportionately concentrated in the same communities (where medical schools are located), factors inflating and depressing the total number of permanent physicians cancel each other out to some extent. The source for the number of physicians is the American Medical Association publication by C.N. Theodore, G. E. Sutter, and E.A. Jokiel (1967), *Distribution of Physicians, Hospitals, and Hospital Beds in the U.S., 1966*, Vol. I, *Regional, State, and County.*

County income and level of urbanization are measured by the annual median family income of county residents in 1959 and the percentage of county residents living in urban areas in 1960. Data for these characteristics are obtained from the U.S. Bureau of the Census (1967) publication based on the 1960 census.[b] However, since the American Medical Association (AMA) publication reports the estimated county population for 1966, this figure is used as the population base for computing the county physician ratio.[c] Relationships are examined for

---

[b]Annual median family is used instead of annual per capita income since the latter may be an unusually high value if there are a few individuals or families in a county with unusually high incomes. Per capita income may thus give a distorted picture of the general economic condition of the county. In most studies, including the study of all counties by Mountin et al. (1942a), per capita income is the measure used.

[c]The population estimates are based on the *Survey of Buying Power*, a publication copyrighted in 1966 by Sales Management, Inc., and reported in C.N. Theordore, G.E. Sutter, and E.A. Jokiel (1967).

counties for 47 contiguous states, with Virginia and the District of Columbia omitted from the analysis. Virginia is eliminated because of the presence of "independent cities" within counties, for which data are reported separately by the census. This leaves a total of 2,971 counties.

The analysis here resembles that of most other studies of the distribution of physicians in that it is concerned with the relationship between the number of physicians per 100,000 population and other characteristics of populations at one point in time: it does not deal with change in the physician ratios over time. Also, no effort is made to estimate the extent to which counties deviate from what would be considered an "adequate" supply of physicians. Since it is apparently impossible to determine the exact number of people most individual physicians are able to serve, and because populations may vary in their need for medical care, the number of physicians per 100,000 necessary to provide adequate care has not been established.[d] However, there is variation among counties— some have higher ratios than others. As in other studies, it is the relationship between variation in the physician ratio and variation in income and urban characteristics that is the focus of study. As noted, the analysis differs from most other studies in the unit of analysis. Most studies have been based on the distribution among regions, states, and metropolitan areas or among counties for selected states and regions. An exception is the early study by Joseph W. Mountin and associates (1942c), in which the distribution of physicians in all United States counties was examined. In some ways the present section might be viewed as a replication of some aspects of that study in that the earlier study investigated the relationship between the physician ratio and county per capita income and proportion of county residents living in areas classified as urban.

It was noted in the previous chapter that 133 counties had no physician in 1971. These counties vary from 200 to 17,400 in total population, and for each of the 133 counties the percentage of urban residents is lower than the percent for the state in which the county is located. In all but 21 counties the 1969 median family income is lower than the corresponding income for the state.[e]

The association of county urban and income characteristics with county physician manpower is not reflected in just these extreme cases, however. The relationship is general. Counties are classified according to level of median family income and percent urban residents: less than $2,000, $2,000-$2,999, $3,000-$3,999, $4,000-$4,999, $5,000-$5,999, and $6,000 and over; and 0.0-9.9%, 10.0-29.9%, 30.0-49.9%, 50.0-69.9%, and 70.0% and over. The average physician ratio is then computed for counties in each income and each urban group. Results for

---

[d]John MacQueen (1968) believes that there is general agreement that a ratio of 100 physicians per 100,000 is sufficient to make medical care readily available for members of a population.

[e]Sources of data: G.A. Roback (1972) and U.S. Bureau of the Census (1971-1972, 1972a).

income are presented in Figure 2-1 and for percent urban in Figure 2-2. (Since income of county is not reported for 13 counties, analysis for income is based on 2,958 counties.)

Income and urban values for each interval are scaled to the midpoint of the counties in the interval, that is, the value midway between the highest and lowest values for counties within the interval. For example, the midpoint for the $2,000-$2,999 range is $2,500.[f] Both figures indicate that each relationship is linear, with the physician ratio increasing continuously throughout the range of income and percentage of urban residents. The figures are based on averages, however, and so may conceal curvilinear patterns, especially at the extremes on the income and urban scales. Comparison of the product-moment correlation

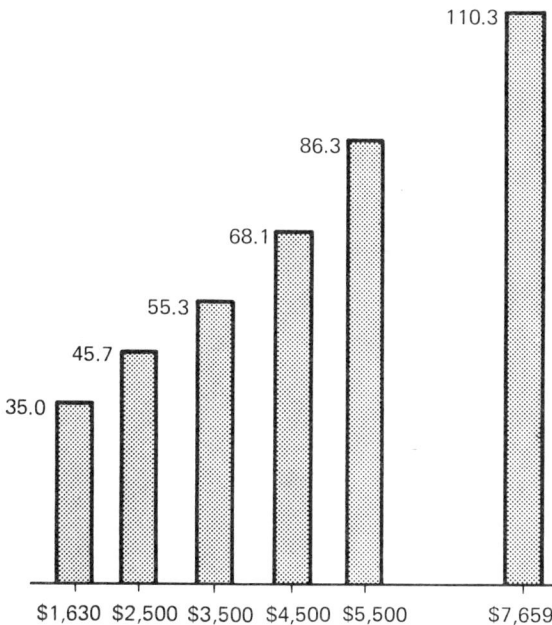

Figure 2-1. Average Number of Physicians per 100,000 Population (1966) for Counties with Different Median Family Income (1966) (2,958 U.S. Counties)

---

[f]The lowest value for counties in the lowest interval and the highest value for counties in the highest interval were obtained from the U.S. Census (1967). Figures indicate that the counties with the lowest and highest median family income in the United States in 1959 had incomes of $1,260 and $9,317. Therefore, the midpoint for the lowest interval is $1,630, and for the highest interval it is $7,659. A similar procedure was followed for percentage urban residents, but since the lowest and highest counties have the lowest and highest values possible (0.0% and 100.0%), the midpoints for counties in the lowest and highest intervals are self-evident.

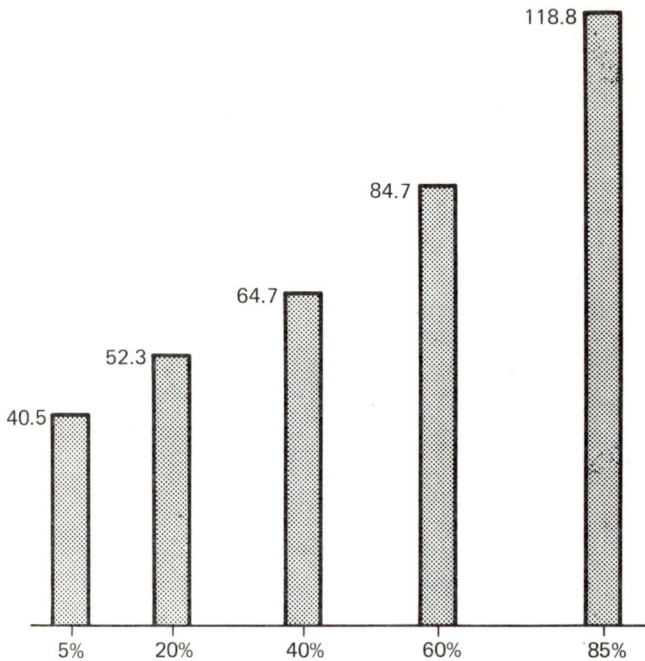

Figure 2-2. Average Number of Physicians per 100,000 Population
(1966) for Counties with Different Percentages of Urban Residents
(1960) (2,971 U.S. Counties)

coefficients and the correlation ratios indicates, however, that the relationships
are basically linear throughout the distributions. The product-moment correlation (r) is a measure of the extent to which two variables are linearly related, the
correlation ratio (η) a measure of the extent to which two variables are related
which takes into account curvilinear trends. The two coefficients are almost
identical for both income and urbanization: for income, $r = 0.38$ and $\eta = 0.39$;
for urbanization $r = 0.45$ and $\eta = 0.46$. The regression coefficients $(b\text{'s})$ are
0.0146 (income) and 0.598 (urbanization). This means that on the average an
increase of $1,000 median family county income increases the number of phy-
sicians per 100,000 county population by 14.6 (0.0146 times 1,000); and an
increase of 10 percent in residents living in urban areas increases the number of

physicians per 100,000 by 5.98 (0.598 times 10). This holds for counties throughout the range of income and urban values. (For a discussion of assumptions in regression analysis as applied to these data, see Appendix B.)

The question arises as to which of the two variables is the most important. Writers do not agree. For example, Joseph W. Mountin, Elliott H. Pennel, and Virginia Nicolay believe that their findings "suggest that consistent population increase [increase in urbanization] in areas reflects factors which serve to attract physicians, but only when the income in these areas is high . . . [Community wealth] is the dominant factor in the maintenance of high physician-population ratios" (1942b, pp. 1942, 1953). Others believe that urban factors are more important. For example, on the basis of the analysis of physician ratios for states, Lee Benham, Alex Maurizi, and Melvin W. Reder conclude that the total effective demand for medical services depends mainly on size of population and secondarily on per capita income; indeed, the "locational preference patterns [of physicians] . . . causes [physician] to sacrifice pecuniary income for the amenities of an urban environment" (1968, p. 345). This conclusion is consistent with that of Rashi Fein and Gerald I. Weber, who contend that the "primary factor affecting the location of new physicians is population change," with states experiencing substantial population increases being better able to attract physicians (Fein and Weber 1971, p. 178). At the same time, Fein and Weber conclude that the determinants of physician location preferences are not altogether clear, but "the one thing that is clear . . . is that the [physician ratio] tends to be highest in those states with the highest per capita income" (Fein and Weber 1971, p. 194). Others contend, however, that "both higher income and urban environment attract more doctors" and that it is impossible to separate their relative effects (Rimlinger and Steele 1963, p. 2).

The latter position would appear to be the most plausible. First, there are theoretical reasons for believing that the two variables are themselves causally interrelated. Both are important in the distribution of physicians but neither exists independently of the other. Consequently, for theoretical reasons it may be unrealistic to try and determine the relative effects of each. These reasons will be outlined in detail in the next chapter. This aside, the fact that income and urban levels of counties are rather highly correlated ($r = 0.59$) makes it difficult to separate their relative effects. The problem is known technically as multicollinearity between independent variables that may make the interpretation of partial correlations dubious. This is so because a very slight variation between each of the independent variables (income and urbanization) and the dependent variable (physician ratio) would give quite different results. Analysis will illustrate.

The zero-order correlation between income and the physician ratio is 0.38, between urbanization and the ratio, 0.45. Since the correlation between income and urbanization is 0.59, the partial correlation for income with urbanization controlled is 0.16 and the correlation for urbanization with income controlled is 0.31. On this basis it might be concluded that the relative effects of urbanization are about twice as great as those of income. But note that the difference between the zero-order correlations is quite small (0.38 to 0.45). Indeed, it would take only a small change for them to be reversed, with 0.38 for urbanization and 0.45 for income. If this were the case, the partial correlation would be exactly opposite to what they are, and the conclusion would be that income is more important than urbanization. Since small differences in correlations can always be expected from one sample to another, a reversal of the two correlations would not be at all unusual in two independent random samples of United States counties. This would be especially the case if there were considerable random measurement error for the variables in question. The implication, therefore, "is that whenever independent variables are highly intercorrelated, it will be necessary to have *both* large samples and accurate measurement" when multiple regression models such as partial correlations are used (Blalock 1972, p. 457). In this particular case, the matter is less problematical than in most studies, since the entire population of counties is included in the analysis (results are not based on a probability sample of American counties) and the measurement error for all three variables is probably quite low. At the same time, analysis based on another year (say, 1974) might yield different results because of relatively minor changes in the location patterns of physicians, through changes either in the pattern of first practice setting or intercommunity migration after that time. Also, there is no doubt some error involved in the measures that might lead to different zero-order correlations for other years even if the actual relationship were exactly the same as that for 1966. Since very small changes could result in substantial differences in the partial correlations, the possibility is not to be dismissed.[g]

The data may be analyzed in a manner that avoids the multicollinear problem. County physician ratios are cross classified in the income and urban categories used in Figures 2-1 and 2-2. For counties in each income-urban category, the median number of physicians in each cell is then computed, as in Table 2-1. (The median is used instead of the mean because the median is not influenced by outlying values, which might be substantial when the number of cases is

---

[g]Some error is undoubtedly involved. It is known that census figures give less than a complete enumeration of the population, with the underreporting of young male blacks being unusually low. Also, there are no doubt some errors in reporting of family income. Moreover, physician data are limited to physicians with known addresses as contained in the AMA Physician Records Service. Nevertheless, given that data are for the total population and that physicians and to some extent the percent urban residents involve only the enumeration of individuals, a minimum of error is no doubt involved. Certainly this would be the case in comparison to most forms of social measurement.

Table 2-1
Median Physician Ratios (1966) for 2,958 U.S. Counties by Median Family Income and Percent Residents Living in Urban Areas

Percent Urban Residents (1960)	Median Family Income (1959)					
	Less Than $2,000	$2,000-$2,999	$3,000-$3,999	$4,000-$4,999	$5,000-$5,999	$6,000 and Over
70.0 and above		33.77 (5)[a]	41.21 (6)	82.01 (58)	105.60 (109)	113.38 (149)
50.0-69.9		43.03 (12)	59.86 (91)	63.30 (146)	76.31 (184)	67.30 (58)
30.0-49.9	43.51 (3)	46.53 (118)	49.44 (175)	50.52 (247)	61.28 (168)	65.30 (25)
10.0-29.9	37.52 (28)	38.43 (124)	44.13 (143)	47.84 (129)	52.80 (57)	38.20 (7)
Less than 10.0	29.64 (81)	29.43 (268)	35.47 (281)	42.06 (206)	46.00 (67)	47.10 (13)

Sources: C.N. Theodore, G.E. Sutter, and E.A. Jokiel (1967) and U.S. Bureau of Census (1967).

[a]Figure in parentheses is number of counties.

small.) Because of the correlation between county income and urbanization, several cells have no counties or too few to provide reliable conclusions (e.g., there are no counties with less than $2,000 and over 69 percent urban residents). In Table 2-1 variation in the physician ratio can be observed across the range of income for counties which are similar with respect to urbanization, and variation in the physician ratio can be observed across the range of urbanization for counties at approximately the same income level. This permits the examination of the effects of each variable while the effects of the other are held constant, or at least restricted to a rather narrow range.

Examination shows that within all urban levels the ratio more or less continuously increases as income level increases and the same is true for the urban variable within each of the income levels. Moreover, the exceptions that do exist are for categories in which the number of counties is quite small and, hence, categories in which the ratio is less apt to be reliable. The really striking thing about Table 2-1 is that the highest values are the high income, high urban group and the lowest values are for low income, low urban group. Results would indicate the following conclusion: To the extent that the economic and urban character of counties are viewed as having separate effects, each has an influence on the distribution of physicians even when the effects of the other are controlled, but that physician manpower is especially high for counties that rank high on both variables and especially low for counties that rank low on both variables. Before discussing a possible explanation for these results, findings for graduates from the class of 1960 are examined.

The Class of 1960

The above relationships are for all physicians as of 1966 and may not be representative of physicians who graduated in more recent years. Data are available for one such class. In 1956 the American Association of Medical Colleges initiated a study, known as the AAMC Longitudinal Study, of 2,821 medical-school freshmen who entered 28 of the 78 four-year United States medical schools in operation at that time.[h] The 78 schools "were stratified according to tax or private support, geographic location, and average intellectual ability level of the student body (as measured by the Medical College Admission Test)," (D'Costa and Yancik 1974, p. 4) so that the 28 schools that were ultimately selected would be representative of all schools with respect to these

---

[h]These data were provided to the author by the American Association of Medical Colleges. (I am most grateful to Dr. Ayres G. D'Costa and Dr. Rosemary Yancik of the American Association of Medical Colleges and officials of the Bureau of Health Services Research and Evaluation of the U.S. Department of Health, Education and Welfare for their assistance in obtaining these data.)

three factors.[i] Students included in the study were asked to complete a questionnaire upon entering medical school in 1950, during their senior year, and in
1965. In addition, these persons were matched with the listing of the American
Medical Association, and data included in the AMA annual questionnaire for
1972 are included in the AAMC data bank. Included in the data are the 1972
addresses of 2,514 of the original 2,821 freshman.[j] From the name of the place
of practice indicated in the address, it was possible to obtain from United States
census publications the name of the county in which the physician was practicing in 1972. It was then possible to determine from census reports the annual
family median income for the county in 1959 and the percentage of county
residents living in urban areas for each county in 1960.[k] Physicians living abroad
and in Virginia, as well as those whose communities could not be located in the
census publications, were eliminated from the analysis. Out of the 2,514 whose
addresses were provided by the AMA, the name and income and percentage of
urban residents for county of practice could be ascertained for 2,418 physicians.[l]

These physicians are cross classified as to the income and urban levels of
their counties of practice. The percentage of physicians in each of several
income-urban combinations is then calculated, as in Table 2-2. In order to convert this percentage to a physician-to-population ratio, the percentage of the
total United States population (1970) living in each of the county income-urban
categories was also computed (with Virginia and District of Columbia eliminated).
The ratio between the percentage of physicians to percentage of population,

---

[i]However, four schools were eliminated and thus "not included in the initial stratification stage of sampling because they drew students from a limited segment of the population.
They are Howard University, Meharry Medical College, Women's Medical College of
Pennsylvania, and College of Medical Evangelists (Loma Linda)." (D'Costa and Yancik,
1974, p. 4). Consequently, the sample is not representative of black and probably female
graduates.

[j]It is believed that the physicians who were not located by the AMA "may have
dropped out of medical education or were missed for some unknown reason such as an
unusual pattern" (D'Costa and Yancik, 1974, p. 6).

[k]Source for county of practice: U.S. Bureau of the Census (1962, 1963). Source of
county income and urban residents: U.S. Bureau of the Census (1967). The reason for
choosing county of practice as the unit of analysis rather than place of practice is due to
the nature of data reported by the Bureau of the Census. The bureau reports only a
limited amount of information for places within counties (e.g., total population), whereas
a number of social, economic, and demographic characteristics are given for counties;
income and urban characteristics are not given for communities within all counties. Consequently, in light of the theoretical framework to be presented in Chapter 3, county
provides the only meaningful unit from the standpoint of available data. However, analysis
is conducted for places of practice within county in Chapter 6 and Chapter 9.

[l]Data are obviously not representative of physicians practicing in Virginia. This is
probably also true for very small communities, since the census does not always list communities by county when the community population is very small.

Table 2-2
Physician-to-Population Ratio by Annual County Median Family Income and Percent of County Residents Living in Urban Areas—Class of 1960 (N = 2,418)

Percent Urban Residents (1960)	Median Family Income (1959)				
	Less Than $5,000	$5,000-$5,999	$6,000-$6,999	$7,000 and Above	Totals
90.0-100.0%	2.15[a] (3.17:1.47)[b]	1.58 (11.08:7.03)	1.35 (17.50:12.93)	1.03 (12.42:12.01)	1.32 (44.17:33.44)
80.0-89.9%	1.61[a] (2.81:1.74)	0.89 (3.89:4.36)	1.25 (6.70:5.52)	1.40 (7.41:5.29)	1.23 (20.81:16.91)
60.0-79.9%	0.59 (2.46:4.14)	0.91 (6.89:7.54)	1.21 (6.83:5.59)	1.38[a] (1.65:1.20)	0.97 (17.83:18.47)
40.0-59.9%	0.56 (3.57:6.32)	0.82 (4.73:5.77)	0.96[a] (2.41:2.52)	——	0.73 (10.71:14.61)
Less than 40.0%	0.29 (3.89:13.27)	0.58[a] (1.61:2.78)	1.88[a] (0.98:0.52)	——	0.39 (6.48:16.57)
Totals	0.59 (15.90:26.94)	1.03 (28.20:27.48)	1.27 (34.42:27.08)	1.16 (21.48:18.54)	1.00 (100.00:100.00)

Sources: AAMC Longitudinal Study and U.S. Bureau of the Census (1967, 1973a).
[a]Denotes low percentage for physician and total population.
[b]Figures are for percentage of physician (1972): percentage of total population (1970).

then, gives a physician-to-population ratio. In Table 2-2 the first figure in parentheses is the percentage of physicians and the second, the percentage of the population. The figure above these is the ratio between the two percentages. This standardizes for population, although results are not presented as the number per 100,000.

The income and urban categories are drawn so as to minimize the number of cells in which the percentages are very low. (As with all United States counties, the correlation between the income and urban levels for this group of physicians is rather high, $r = 0.45$.) Consequently, the categories are drawn differently from those in Table 2-1. Moreover, the ratios in the two tables are obtained by different procedures. The results in Table 2-1 are obtained by first computing the physician-to-population ratio for *each* of 2,958 counties and then getting the median ratio for counties in each income and urban level. Therefore, results in Table 2-1 are based on measures for counties. The ratios in Table 2-2 are for the number of physicians in all counties within an income or urban interval to the total population for all counties in the interval; hence, the ratio for each cell is for the aggregate of all physicians to total population for all counties of certain income and urban intervals and not the median physician-to-population ratio for counties within those intervals. Therefore, if the ratio in Table 2-2 is 1.00, it means that the percentage of the 2,418 physicians who practice in counties in that cell is the same percentage as the total population who live in those counties. For example, the cell in the lower left corner of Table 2-2 shows that 3.89 percent of the physicians practice in counties with less than $5,000 median family income and less than 40.0 percent urban residents but that 13.27 percent of the total population live in such counties. The resulting physician:total population ratio is 0.29, which means that the section of the population living in these counties got only 29 percent of its proportionate share of physicians from the class of 1960, based on its share of the total 1970 population. In contrast, the population in counties with $7,000 annual family income and above and over 90.0 percent urban residents got 103 percent of its share.

Two types of comparisons are to be made in Table 2-2. The first comparisons are between the ratios in the totals column and row. The totals column gives the physician-to-population ratio by urban level; as can be seen the ratio increases continuously as urbanization increases. The row totals indicate that the ratio also increases as income level increases, although the relationship is not linear since the ratio for the highest income level is slightly lower than that for the next highest income level. Although the analysis here is not exactly comparable to that of the previous section, the similarity between these relationships and those depicted in Figures 2-1 and 2-2 is clear. Consequently, the 1960 graduating class would appear to be representative of the population of United States physicians with respect to the relationships between physician manpower and county income and urbanization.

At the same time, other comparisons indicate that the effects of income and urbanization are different from those indicated in Table 2-1. Comparing the effect of urbanization within the columns of Table 2-2 reveals that the ratios increase as urbanization increases for the two lowest income levels and, if cells with low percentages are ignored, increases slightly with urbanization for counties in the $6,000-$6,999 range and then tends to decrease for the highest income interval. Within row comparison shows that the ratio increases as income increases for the urban levels below 90.0 percent and decreases as income decreases for the highest urban level. This indicates, then, that at least for the class of 1960, income and urbanization interact. The relationship of each to the physician ratio is not constant but varies depending on the value of the other. Specifically, the positive effects of each are greatest when the values of the other are lowest, and are actually negative when the values of the other are highest. Comparison of Table 2-2 with 2-1 suggests that this particular pattern is more typical of more recent graduates than of all physicians.[m]

Nevertheless, the totals columns and rows for the two tables are striking in their similarity. The distribution of physician graduates of 1960 is thus both similar to and different from the distribution of all physicians.

Discussion

Results indicate two general patterns. Findings for all counties and for the class of 1960 reveal that both income and urbanization are related to physician manpower. This is consistent with the results of most other studies of larger geographical units as well as with much public opinion. They are also consistent with the earlier study of Mountin and associates, and thus indicate that the maldistribution of physicians in counties of different income and urban levels today follows a pattern that has existed for at least a half-century. Results for the class of 1960 suggest, however, that a new pattern has emerged in which income and urbanization interact. An interpretation of the distribution of physician manpower in terms of income and urban characteristics must account for both patterns.

A common interpretation of the maldistribution of physicians is in terms of individual characteristics of physicians. For example, some view the maldistribution as stemming from the business orientation of physicians (cf. Kaplan 1970) or

---

[m]It is tempting to combine the income and urban county levels for the class of 1960 to form a single scale. Although this would make for a more parsimonious treatment of the data, it would conceal the interaction effects in Table 2-2 as well as important differences between counties of different income and urban levels in the production of physicians and recruitment-production ratios, which will be examined in subsequent chapters.

their monetary motives (Steele and Rimlinger 1967).[n] Such a view is consistent with the first pattern, particularly those for county income. In general, counties with high income provide more opportunities than counties with low income to enhance physician income. Such an interpretation is not without its problems, however.

First, a number of things are reflected by the income index, such as cultural diversity, institutions that provide more attractive recreational and leisure-time activity, better quality educational institutions for children, and access to more medical facilities and to more medical colleagues—all of which have been cited as factors in community differences in physician manpower (American Medical Association 1973, pp. 29-65). In addition, location in economically depressed rural communities may offer greater economic opportunity per se than more affluent urban communities. Indeed, one of the reasons physicians apparently choose to begin practicing in a small community is the advantage it offers in developing a thriving practice early (Parker and Tuxhill 1967). And the results of one study show that the incomes of physicians in rural Southern Appalachian communities compare favorably with those of nonrural physicians in the region (Champion and Olsen 1971). (It is also true that in this study physicians were not aware of this; consequently, it may not have influenced where they decided to practice.) Nevertheless, it is probable that purely economic motivation is reflected to some extent in the results. All other things being equal, physicians are probably disposed to locate in counties with higher income levels because these counties promise to offer the most in the way of economic opportunity.

The urban index also reflects many of the same factors reflected in the income index. In addition, it reflects factors which refer to an "external economy of scale," which is a major factor in the location of most types of industry. The economies provided by the clustering of people (level of urbanization) is probably more important in the service industry than other industries. In extractive industries, for example, economies are realized from the *dispersal* of the population because of the diminishing returns associated with intensive (rather than extensive) cultivation and extraction which high population concentration would require. On the other hand, manufacturing industries usually experience a much longer state of increasing returns with greater concentration. Even so, manufacturers may find it more economical to locate so as to minimize the transportation

---

[n]Even interpretations that emphasize the roles of the American Medical Association and medical schools may tend to focus on motivational factors. For example, the restriction of the supply of physicians, which some view as a major reason for the maldistribution and the result of policies of both the American Medical Association and medical schools, is frequently viewed as motivated by economic considerations.

of material and distribution of products, the cost of which the producer has to
bear, at the expense of transportation for workers (job commuting), which
the workers have to bear. Service industries also experience increasing returns
with concentration, but need also

> to weigh the costs of movement of both the producer (lawyer, doctor,
> teacher) and the consumer (client, patient, student), although these
> are sometimes substitutive (the housecall). A dense cluster of people—
> a city—is almost by definition a physical manifestation of a planned
> arrangement for the heavy physical interaction especially characteristic
> of the service industries (Thompson 1969, p. 12).

Thus, physicians like providers of most services, especially if they are self-
employed, want to locate so as to have convenient access to as many potential
clients (patients) as possible. Consequently, location in areas of large *and*
dense populations are desirable. A large county population may itself not be
desirable because the population may be widely scattered, whereas a dense
population in a very small county may not be particularly desirable because
the number of persons is so small. The proportion of residents classified as
residing in urban areas, which is the index of "urbanization" used in this and
most other studies, is a close approximation to the combination of county size
and density. The percentage of persons living in urban areas includes

> all persons living in (a) places of 2,500 inhabitants or more incorporated
> as cities, boroughs, villages, and towns (except towns in New England,
> New York, and Wisconsin); (b) the densely settled urban fringe, whether
> incorporated or unincorporated, of urbanized areas; (c) towns in New
> England and townships in New Jersey and Pennsylvania which contain
> no incorporated municipalities as subdivisions and which have either
> 25,000 inhabitants or more, or a population of 2,500 to 25,000 and a
> density of 1,500 persons or more per square mile; (d) counties in States
> other than the New England states, New Jersey, and Pennsylvania that
> have no incorporated municipalities within their boundaries and have a
> density of 1,500 persons or more per square mile; and (3) unincorpo-
> rated places of 2,500 inhabitants or more (U.S. Bureau of the Census
> 1967, p. xx).

The size-density of a population in itself—aside from cultural and social factors
that are correlated with it—probably exerts an influence on physician locations
because of the "external economies of scale" it provides.[o]

––––––––––––––––––

[o]It is because the census definition of urban more closely approximates the conception of an external scale for physicians that it is used rather than the population density

Although there are alternative motivational explanations besides economic factors for the relationships between the physician-to-population ratio and county income and urban levels, this is not in my view the chief limitation of the approach. The primary limitation is that the approach focuses only on one side of the relationship—the supply side. It takes the "demand characteristics" of communities as given, and then accounts for the supply of physicians in terms of those characteristics, via the motives of physicians. Missing is an explanation for the demand characteristics themselves. This is true for all motivational explanations and not just those that emphasize economic elements. Even if the results were due to county differences in medical facilities that motivate physicians for professional reasons, an explanation of why county income (urbanization) and hospital facilities are related would be required.[P]

In summary, characteristics of communities that serve to attract physicians are themselves the result of forces that need to be identified and taken into account. Consequently, rather than seeking an explanation of the distribution of physicians in terms of motives—economic, professional, cultural or otherwise—an equally fruitful approach might be one that focuses on community and on providing an explanation for the relationships between structural characteristics of communities. Motivational frameworks that account for why physicians locate where they do need to be complemented with frameworks that deal with causal relationships between characteristics of communities. And this framework must account for the two patterns described in this chapter. The major elements of such a framework are presented in the next chapter.

(e.g., number of persons per square mile). Only if population density and the total population are highly correlated would density or total population provide a measure that reflects both the total population and the clustering (or density) of the population. The product-moment correlation between total population and persons per square mile for the 2,978 United States counties is only 0.41. Population size would constitute a measure of size and density when units (counties) are equal in area size.

[P]The relationship of hospitals and medical schools to the physician ratio as well as to county income and urbanization is investigated in chapters 10 and 11.

3 A Framework of Community and a Causal Interpretation

A basic difference between motivational frameworks and the one presented in this chapter is in the unit of analysis. In motivational frameworks the individual is the unit of analysis, whereas in the one presented here, the community is. With communities as the units of analysis, the physician-to-population ratio is viewed as a property of community and as causally related to other properties of community. Causal interpretations of county physician ratios are in terms of characteristics of communities, and even characteristics that extend beyond single communities, rather than in terms of factors that motivate physicians to locate their practices in some communities rather than others. Therefore, in contrast to frameworks that focus on explaining why physicians tend to locate in communities with certain characteristics rather than others, effort here focuses on explaining community differences in the characteristics themselves (including the physician ratio) and the relationships among the characteristics. As will be seen, however, the framework presented is not an alternative to frameworks that focus on individual characteristics of physicians so much as it serves to complement those frameworks.

It goes without saying that any causal framework for the distribution of physicians, or for any other occupational group, is an oversimplification of a complex phenomenon. Probably no logically consistent framework could include all the factors that are correlated with physician ratios and that exert a causal influence on the distribution of physicians. In the development of the framework presented here the focus is on the patterns observed in the previous chapter. In addition, however, the framework provides a guide for the analysis and interpretation in subsequent chapters concerning community differences in the production of physicians; the role of specialization, hospitals, and medical schools in the distribution of physicians; the effect of suburbanization; the persistence of the maldistribution inspite of efforts to reduce the severity of the problem; and for assessing the actual or potential impact of various public policy programs.

Causal statements were implied, of course, in the previous chapter. In the relationship between income (urban) level of counties and the physician ratio, income (urban) level of county was viewed as causing the physician ratio rather than the reverse. The effort in this chapter is to extend such statements by viewing these causal relationships within a more general system of causal relationships.

Although community is the focus of the framework, in no sense should the system of causal relationships presented be viewed as a fully developed general theory of community. Existing data are too limited and existing theoretical ideas of community too fragmentary to permit the development of such a theory.[a] Consequently, the ideas presented in this chapter are viewed more as a bare outline and the fragments that a well-developed theory would incorporate. It will, however, provide a general framework for interpreting aspects of the maldistribution of physicians.

Since so much of the empirical analysis in this book is for county units, a few comments are in order concerning the theoretical statement and the empirical results that bear on that statement. Counties are not infrequently viewed as important primarily for political administrative reasons, and the fact that so much census data exist by county is a consequence of this. Therefore, data on counties are often viewed as of quite limited value because counties do not correspond to circumscribed cultural, social and economic areas. It is difficult to refute this argument, if for no other reason than the difficulty involved in identifying the boundaries of a large number of different cultural, social and economic areas. Nevertheless, while it is true that counties are not coterminous with cultural, social, and economic areas, the fact that they are political and administrative units makes them the locus of much economic, social, and cultural activity. School systems, law enforcement systems, medical associations and various other institutions are countywide in scope, and efforts to attract industry and business are frequently led by representatives of the entire county and not by representatives of some small areas within the county. Thus, although counties are not perfect reflections of the concept of community, as this term is used in so much of the sociological literature (cf. Warren 1972), the correspondence is close enough to refer to counties as communities.[b]

Traditionally in sociology, conceptualizations of community have tended to view communities as self-contained social units separated from the rest of the world. Writers have noted that this may give an erroneous view of communities, since so much of what happens within the community is causally related to events outside the community (cf. Martindale and Hanson 1969; Warren 1972; Zentner 1973). It seems useful, therefore, to distinguish between the local community context and the more inclusive context of which the community is a part. Physician manpower of counties is viewed within these contexts.

The Local Community as Context

The local context of medical care in American communities includes a wide

---

[a]For an overview, see Roland L. Warren (1972).

[b]For an analysis which makes a case for treating counting as meaningful units of analysis, see G. Edward Stephen (1971).

number of factors and would include differences in community culture as well as differences in political, economic, and social institutions. While there is an important truth here—any institution is only one part of a community and is a reflection of other aspects of those broader systems, it does not help us very much. It is difficult to conceptualize everything about a community as a cultural, political, economic, and social phenomenon that at the same time guides the construction of measures that will permit distinctions between communities. As in all theoretical frameworks, a framework of community must be selective in its focus.

The contextual properties of characteristics of community that have received attention from sociologists vary. Some view community primarily in terms of its power structure (e.g., Hunter 1953), some in terms of cleavage and conflict between factions in the community (e.g., Coleman 1959); others view it as a system of social stratification (e.g., Warner 1959), and still others view it in terms of a system of social interaction (e.g., Kaufman 1959). None is more valid than the other: All communities have power structures, conflicts between individuals and groups, a system of socioeconomic classes, and networks of social interaction. Different points of reference, however, are more useful for some purposes than others. If one wishes to know how and who makes major decisions in communities, a focus on power structure is probably the most fruitful approach, while if one wishes to distinguish between styles of life and the differential distribution of income and privilege, studies of communities in terms of a system of social stratification will usually yield better results.

Many sociological studies of community have been limited to the study of single communities and have focused on showing how some aspect of a community is part of the broader community context, however viewed. Such studies are limited in that it is not always possible to know to what extent the events that are believed to be linked to the broader community context are in fact closely linked to it. This is so because the context is not a variable quality since only one community is the object of study. Therefore, it is hard to know whether differences in the factors explained in terms of the community context are in fact related to differences in community context (see Reiss 1954 and 1966). In our case, for example, it is necessary to understand how community differences in the supply of physicians is related to differences in general contextual properties of communities.

A number of approaches for classifying communities in terms of general properties is based on the idea of economic base. In some formulations this is viewed primarily in terms of export economic base (e.g., industry), which gives the community market power and something to exchange with the rest of society. In general, however, there is a lack of agreement as to how community economic base is to be specifically defined and delineated (e.g., in terms of employment structure, income flows, or values added in production) (Duncan et al. 1960, p. 33). Rather than attempt to identify the specific properties of the economic base that are most important, the conception and definition of economic base here is more global. Regardless of the precise base, communities differ with respect to overall economic welfare. This is reflected in the earlier measure of county wealth—median family income, "since the level of income is the single most meaningful measure of [a community's] economic welfare" (Thompson 1969, p. 12). At the most general level it is an index of the strength of community economic institutions regardless of the precise nature of those institutions (e.g., durable manufacturing, extractive industry, etc.).

An increase in the strength of local economic institutions provides jobs, attracts labor, and increases the community population base. These, in turn, increase the local tax base, and in time lead to an increase in the occupational skill mix and educational level of the community; research institutions and vocational and technical schools frequently develop in the area and the growth of colleges and universities may be encouraged. Growth in the economic base and population base, then, leads to growth in the local occupational-service sector. In time this sector may become the major asset of the community, attracting industries that require sophisticated skill and, incidentally, workers who can command high incomes, thus strengthening the overall economic base and increasing community income even further. Over the long run, then, it is difficult to know what leads to what—economic base to the occupational-service sector or vice versa (Thompson 1967, p. 8). The essential point is that in the long run the two are mutually dependent. A locality with a new industry might

> come in time to acquire the education and skill which merits a relative high local wage rate. High wage rates, however acquired, provide the personal income and tax base needed to build superior social overhead and thereby to provide a wholly new *economic* base to support new *export bases*. [Although this may lead to a labor market that is too expensive for many industries], by the time the moment of truth arrives, the local labor force could have matured in education and skill to the point where it is no longer significantly overpriced, and has become, in fact, a scarce factor and the principle local attraction.

> Thus, in this case, no equilibrating force would ever come into play. The original nexus of market power could lead, instead, to a set of disequilibrating forces, as [market] power leads to affluence, and affluence leads to education and skill, and so on to further affluence (Thompson 1969, p. 15; author's emphasis).

Community population base and community wealth are also mutually dependent. Large populations make communities attractive to industrial firms because of the external economies they provide in the form of convenient access to transporation networks, proximity to many suppliers and buyers, the presence of a large labor force, and the ability to locate in one place many diverse aspects of manufacturing operations that require large numbers of employees, hence facilitating communication and coordination between different operations. The economies of scale associated with large numbers tend to override such social and psychological dis-economies of congestion, pollution, and the cost of transportation to employees and the general public.[c] Such economies in turn attract more industry, thus strengthening the economic base, which strengthens the local occupational-service structure, and so on in a circle.

By the same token, the concentration of large numbers of individuals in a locality tends to encourage the development of aspects of the local occupational-service sector, such as the medical, legal, pharmaceutical, and other professions that provide direct services to the public. And, of course, the presence of a strong occupational-service sector helps to make the community attractive and, hence, helps to attract a larger population.

In summary, community economic base, population, and the occupational-service sector are interdependent. Change in one is apt to result in changes in the other two. It is within the context of these three interrelated aspects of communities that the local supply of physician manpower, which is only one component of the local occupational-service sector, is viewed. An implication is that the relationships of the physician ratio to community wealth and urbanization should be similar to the corresponding relationships for other occupations making up the service sector. Before investigating the matter empirically, a discussion of the extracommunity context is presented.

The Extra Community Context

In their study of metropolitan communities in the United States, Duncan et al. state that "to understand metropolitan communities we must examine them in the context of a more inclusive system" (Duncan et al. 1960, p. 4). They believe that it is useful to view this context in terms of hierarchy. They state: "The hierarchy concept . . . assumes or implies that a collection of cities, if properly delimited, may be regarded as a *system*. The investigator undertaking comparative urban research with the concept of system of cities in mind will be interested in properties of the system as such rather than merely the varying traits of individual cities" (Duncan et al. 1960, p. 6). In the current framework the collection of counties are viewed more accurately in terms of a rank system rather than a hierarchic system. Counties are viewed as arranged in rank order

---

[c]Wilbur R. Thompson also argues that the classic factors of production—entrepreneurship, capital, labor and land—all tend to maintain the growth of larger communities rather than to revitalize smaller communities (Thompson 1969, pp. 9-12).

that possesses a systemic property. Therefore, interest is not limited to the economy, population, services sector and physician manpower of individual counties and the fact that counties vary with respect to these properties. Interest is in how counties and their traits are part of a system that extends beyond the boundaries of individual counties.

Two problems must be resolved in viewing counties in terms of a rank system. One, of course, is the identification of variables that differentiate between counties and of the hierarchic relationships between counties in terms of those variables. The other is the identification of the systemic properties that regulate the relationships between the variables. The solution of both of these problems depends on the development of a unified theory of community. Since there is no such theory, proposals that attempt to solve these problems must be presented as tentative. It is in this spirit that the following remarks are offered.

As to the first problem, it has been suggested that it is useful to view communities in terms of the variables of economic base, population base, and local occupational-service structure. Median family income of county was presented as a measure of economic base. A measure of population is problematical because of the concept of external economies, which requires that the population be concentrated as well as large. The proportion of residents classified as residing in urban areas is a rough approximation to this (see pp. 30 above). For a measure of the local occupational-service sector, the proportion of all employed males classified by the census in "professional, technical and kindred" occupations is used.[d] Occupations included in this category are accountants, architects, engineers, dentists, lawyers, pharmacists, teachers, and veterinarians, as well as physicians. Not all occupations included are truly professional, however, in the sense that they normally require advanced educational and occupational training. For example, athletes, dancers, musicians, and dental and medical technicians are included. In general, however, from among the approximately 500 detailed occupational categories listed by the U.S. Census, those included in the "professional and kindred" category represent occupations that require the most education and skill. In comparison with a median of 11.1 years completed for all the experienced labor force in 1960, the median for professional and technical workers was 16.3. The nearest major occupational category to professional and kindred workers is "managers, officials and proprietors," which had a median of 12.5 years (U.S. Bureau of the Census 1963). Therefore, the proportion of all employed males who are classified in the professional and technical category is used to index the county occupational skill mix or local service sector. It is referred to as the "professional ratio."

_____

[d]Source of data is U.S. Bureau of the Census (1962-1963). Data are limited to males because of the need to compare the distribution of all professional, technical and kindred occupations with the distribution of physicians, and 93 percent of physicians in 1967 were male (Theodore, Sutter, and Haug 1968, p. 9).

According to the formulation above, relationships between county wealth, urban residents, and the professional ratio would be expected. The product-moment correlation coefficients are 0.58 and 0.51 between community wealth and the urban and professional ratios respectively, and 0.44 between the urban and professional ratios.[e] Even allowing for attenuation due to errors of measurement, the correlations are far from 1.00, though high by sociological standards. The less than perfect correlations reflect the fact that each of the above three factors are due to factors besides the other two. (The magnitudes of the correlations are not reduced by curvilinear patterns, since the correlation ratios for the relationships between the professional ratio and income and urbanization are 0.52 and 0.45, which are almost identical to the product-moment correlations.) For example, community wealth may result from the discovery of mineral deposits or massive federal spending (e.g., Oak Ridge, Huntsville) but a large dense population may not materialize (although an increase may occur, it is not proportionate to the increase in wealth). A large population may be attracted to areas because of certain climatic and scenic qualities and not because occupational opportunities are plentiful, as in the case of communities in Florida and Arizona, many of which have a large proportion of retired persons. Professional persons may be influenced by the quality of life offered by a community as well as economic aspects and the external economies of scale provided by the composition of its population. Also, size of total population and its racial-ethnic composition are not considered. In addition, the analysis assumes that counties are homogeneous units and clearly differentiated from other counties in economic pattern and demographic and occupational structures. The assumption is obviously not true for all counties; for most counties the assumption is probably true only in part.

The analysis also assumes that all counties of the United States constitute a national system. Obviously, the assumption is not completely valid, certainly not in the short run. Changes in the economic base, population, and occupational service sector in a county in the northwestern part of Washington has no immediate impact on the corresponding sectors in the southern part of Florida. The assumption is probably more valid on a regional basis. Separate analysis for each of the nine census regions reveals that the correlations are about the same for all nine regions of the country (see Table 3-1). With the exception of the two correlations for the professional ratio in the West North Central region, correlations are moderate to high in magnitude. Even within this region, analysis for each of the states separately indicates that with the exception of one state (Missouri) the magnitudes of the correlations for the professional ratio are moderate to high;

---

[e]Comparison of the results for the urban index with measures of total county population and of population per square mile for all United States counties proves interesting. For income, the r's are 0.33 and 0.12 for total population and population density in comparison to 0.58 for percentage of urban residents. The correlations between the professional ratio and total population and density are 0.24 and 0.09, in comparison to 0.44 between the professional ratio and the urban index.

Table 3-1
Product-Moment Correlations Between County Family Median Income (1959),
Percent County Residents Living in Urban Areas (1960), and County
Professional Ratio (1960)–by Region

Region	Income and Urban	Income and Professional Ratio	Urban and Professional Ratio	N[a]
New England	0.72	0.80	0.54	67
Middle Atlantic	0.70	0.75	0.46	150
East North Central	0.72	0.58	0.54	436
West North Central	0.68	0.18	0.22	619
South Atlantic	0.62	0.65	0.47	454
East South Central	0.69	0.55	0.55	364
West South Central	0.50	0.44	0.50	470
Rocky Mountain	0.46	0.47	0.48	278
Pacific Coast	0.52	0.46	0.37	133

Source: U.S. Bureau of the Census (1962, 1963; 1967) and C.N. Theodore, G.E. Sutter, and E.A. Jokiel (1967).

[a]N is number of counties. In some regions the correlations for income are based on a slightly lower figure because in 13 counties median family income is not reported.

the average correlation between median income and the professional ratio for this region with Missouri excluded is 0.53, and the average for percentage of urban residents and the professional ratio is 0.58. Overall, then, results are consistent with the formulation that the three variables are arranged in a system of ranks, in that county position on one variable tends to correspond to its position on another.

Problems with the analysis are to be noted, however. The income index and the professional ratio are not entirely independent of each other. Since professional and technical workers contribute to community income, and because their incomes are higher on the average than those of other workers except managers, officials, and proprietors, a proportionate increase in professional and technical workers in a county raises the median family income of the county. At the same time, however, only 10.3 percent of the United States employed labor force were in professional and technical occupations in 1960 (U.S. Bureau of the Census 1963a, pp. 1-2). Consequently, the results do show to a substantial degree the relationship between the general wealth of a community and the professional ratio. There is no such problem with the relationships involving the percent of urban residents, and the correlations are substantial in magnitude.[f]

The System Property

As noted, it is unrealistic to view communities as self-contained units. They are best viewed in terms of their relationship to other communities and to the larger society. The results above are consistent with this view. They indicate that there are indeed statistical relationships between counties, and in this sense results are consistent with the idea that the individual counties are part of a rank system that is external to individual counties and that provides a more inclusive context within which individual counties may be viewed. However, results do not indicate how the relationships are the product of a characteristic of this system. They do not reveal how county position on the three variables is influenced by a property of the system.

The principle by which a community property is influenced by the system context beyond the community may be illustrated by Roland Warren's observation that local communities have become increasingly dependent on "extra-community systems" so that the relationship "of community units to state and national systems" has been strengthened (Warren, 1972, p. 52). Consequently, what happens to agencies and institutions in an individual community is as much a function of what happens in the wider system as what happens at the local level. For example, the local post offices, American Legion posts, churches, chain grocery and department stores, labor union locals, school systems, industrial plants—all are part of regional or national systems and are controlled and regulated at points outside the community (Warren, 1972, pp. 53-94). Consequently, local communities do not have control over some of their local institutions because those institutions are part of a broader context and many local institutions can be understood only with reference to that broader context.

It is not likely that the results in Table 3-1 are due to the kind of system-wide planning that Warren observes, such as in the United States postal system.

---

[f]However, there is another problem with the urban index as it is related to the professional ratio. The urban and professional ratios have denominators that, while not the same, may be highly correlated (the denominator of the professional ratio—total number of males in the labor force—is probably correlated with the denominator of the urban index—the total population). The problem is discussed in Appendix A. Considering the nature of the data there is little that can be done other than note the existence of these problems. It is better to proceed to develop theory on the basis of data that are less than perfect than to wait until data and resulting measures have been perfected. If the latter course were adopted, one may well wait forever.

More likely, they stem from the fact that each variable, which is itself the result of a number of units (industries, occupations, individuals) making separate location decisions, has a causal effect on the other two. Industries with the best paying jobs tend to move to communities that have population bases which permit important external economies and where the occupational skills are high, thus contributing to the intercorrelations between community wealth, size-density, and the local occupational-service sector (skill mix). And the over-all population and persons with technical occupational skills tend to move to communities where the well-paying jobs are to be found, and this also contributes to the interrelations. The process is not planned at one central location; "planning" is done by many separate industries and individuals who make independent locational decisions. The aggregate of the many decisions lead to the patterns observed in Table 3-1. For whatever reason—central location, proximity to transportation networks (waterways, railroads, highways, etc.), massive federal spending, availability of natural resources (e.g., coal, water power, etc.)—certain communities are able to attract industry and raise their income level. This leads to a strong local occupational-service sector, which helps to maintain the local income level as well as to attract additional industry, population, and persons with high-level educations and occupational skills.

New industries are the highest growth industries and they also require the use of sophisticated skills; in consequence, they pay higher wages and salaries. Because these industries need sophisticated occupational skills and technical expertise, they tend to locate in communities where those resources exist. At the same time, the older and slower growing industries, in which jobs have become highly routinized, may require less skill and expertise; hence, they tend to move to communities where the occupational skills and educational levels are lower and, therefore, where wage rates are lower. Wilbur R. Thompson states (1969, pp. 8-9):

> In national perspective, industries filter down through the system of cities, from places of greater to lesser industrial sophistication. Most often the highest skills are needed in the difficult, early stage of mastering a new process, and skill requirements decline steadily as the production process is rationalized and routinized with experience. As the industry slides down the learning curve, the high wage rates of the most industrially sophisticated innovating areas become superfluous. The aging industry seeks out industrial backwaters where the cheaper labor is now up to the lessened demands of the simplified process . . . In the long run, the larger, more sophisticated urban economies can . . . continue to earn above-average incomes only by continually performing the more difficult work.

A filter-down theory of industrial location would go far toward explaining the isolated small town's lament that it always gets the slow-growing industries. They find they must run to stand still, as their industrial catches seem only to come to these out-of-the-way places to die. These smaller, industrial novices also struggle to raise per capita income over the hurdle of industries which pay the lowest wage rates. Clearly, the twin characteristics of slow growth and low wage rates (low skills) might be viewed as two facets of the aging industry. The smaller, less industrially advanced area struggles to achieve an average rate of growth out of enlarging shares of slow-growing industries, which were attracted by the area's low wage rates. It would seem, then, that both the larger industrial centers from which, and the smaller areas to which, industries filter down must run to stand still (at the national average growth rate); the larger areas do, however, run for higher stakes.

Moreover, because of the low level skills possessed by workers of many communities, the wage rate for comparable work may be lower than in other communities. In the study of an economically declining community, Don Martindale and R. Galen Hanson observe: "As farmers are pressed off the land in the towns, they may form local enclaves of labor that may be exploited more cheaply than the labor of the larger urban centers by . . . industrial concerns" (1969, p. 109). In any case, since a community's wealth and the strength of its occupational-service sector are causally related, communities that have industries with low wage rates are apt also to have weaker occupational-service sectors, and vice versa, and this will usually mean a low supply of physicians.

At the same time, communities with stronger economies and local service sectors do not always retain their advantage over other communities. Just as individuals drop and rise in economic status, so communities rise and fall. Wealthy communities have been known to decline and not all currently wealthy communities were always affluent. For example, a sharp and sudden decrease in the demand for the product of a community's major industry may lead to a decline in community income because the change occurs before the industy has had an opportunity to adapt to changing conditions (e.g., by diversifying). Also, the rapid growth of the local service sector, which consists of persons with technical occupational skills as well as the service professions, may make labor too expensive for new industry as well as for the original industry that led to a high skill sector in the first place. Or strong labor unions may require production standards that are not in line with new technological processes that permit increases in productivity, so that the industry chooses to locate elsewhere (Thompson 1969, p. 4). Although such changes may occur dramatically, they usually occur over the long run rather than the short run; just as upward and downward mobility are rare for individuals and occur in short steps rather than long leaps, changes in the social and economic institutions of communities are slow. The fact that a strong economic base, strong occupational-service sector, ability to attract persons with talent and skill from less advantaged communities, and large populations with their external economies of scale tend to go together and are mutually dependent is a constraint on rapid change. It usually allows wealthier communities to maintain their advantages over time and constrains poorer communities to live with the disadvantages they have inherited from the past.

This may be illustrated with the relationship between county wealth (as indexed by median family income in 1959) and growth in the population for counties from 1950 to 1970. In general, the relative ordering of counties on population in 1970 was about the same as in 1950, as indicated by the r of 0.95 between them; thus, the best prediction for the rank of a county's population in 1970 is its rank in 1950. Consequently, in showing the extent to which community wealth had any effect on the changes that did occur in this 20-year period, it will be necessary to control for population in 1950. The partial correlation between 1970 population and 1960 median family income with 1950 population controlled is 0.21.[g] Thus, although there was very little change in the relative differences between counties in population in 1970 and 1950, the change that did occur was associated with community income. The wealthier communities grew more, but not much more.

In summary, the formulation views communities in terms of the interdependencies between economic, population and occupational-service sector. Change in one is influenced by change in the other; and by the same token, efforts to change one aspect of community are constrained if change does not occur in the others. The processes that create the ranking of counties tend to perpetuate the ranking through time. Newer industries with higher pay scales move to communities in which higher-paying industries are already located because of the external economies and skilled labor services such communities provide. And as a result, the more educated and skilled persons from economically deprived areas are apt to be attracted to more densely populated and wealthier communities because occupational opportunities provided by industry are greater in such communities. Thus, efforts to improve the educational and occupational skill mix in depressed areas in order to attract industry tend not to improve the local economic situation at all: residents who acquire the education and skills tend to more to the already more prosperous communities where occupational and economic opportunities as well as cultural and social advantages are more plentiful (cf. Hansen 1970). The tendency for the more affluent and less affluent communities to remain in their relative positions over time is, therefore, reinforced by migration patterns.

---

[g]The zero-order correlations between median family income in 1959 and total population are 0.28 (for 1950 population) and 0.33 (for 1970 population). Sources of data are U.S. Bureau of Census (1952-1953, 1967, and 1973a).

Implications of the Framework

Although the framework is crude and measures of variables used to illustrate various aspects of it are less than perfect, it is consistent with the results of the previous chapter. It also provides a general orientation for examining results and assessing policy programs in later chapters. In the remainder of this chapter two implications of the framework are examined. The first concerns the similarity between the distribution of physicians and other occupational groups; the other concerns changes in the distribution of physicians.

Physicians and other Professional Occupations

According to the formulation, physicians, as a component of the local occupational-service sector, should be related to community income and urbanization much as the professional ratio is. The product-moment correlation coefficients are 0.51 and 0.44 between this ratio and community wealth and percent urban, which compare with the corresponding correlations for the physician ratio, 0.39 and 0.46.[h] More revealing is the comparison of the slope of the regression lines of the two ratios on county income and percent urban.

Figure 3-1 gives the regression coefficients for both ratios on median family income. The regression coefficients (*b*'s) must be interpreted somewhat differently in the two cases because the denominators differ. For the physician ratio, the *b* of 0.0158 indicates that, on the average, an increase of $1,000 median family income will result in an increase of 15.8 physicians per 100,000 total population. In the case of all professionals, the *b* of 0.0146 means that as median family income increases by $1,000, the number of males in the labor force who are in professional and technical occupations increases on the average by 14.6 persons per 1,000 males in the labor force. Comparison of the two regression lines indicate that although the slope for the physician ratio is slightly steeper, the resemblance of the two slopes is clear. The distribution of physicians appears indeed to be part of a more general distributional pattern.[i]

---

[h]Note again that the physician ratio and the professional ratio have denominators that, while not identical, are probably highly correlated (total population for the physician ratio and total male labor force for the professional ratio). The reader again is referred to Appendix A for a discussion of the problem.

[i]There is a technical problem in making the comparison between regression slopes in Figure 3-1. When the same independent variable is included in different regression analyses, the magnitude of the regression coefficient will vary depending on variation in the dependent variable. Since in this case the independent variable is the same (median family income), differences in the magnitude of the regression coefficient will be influenced

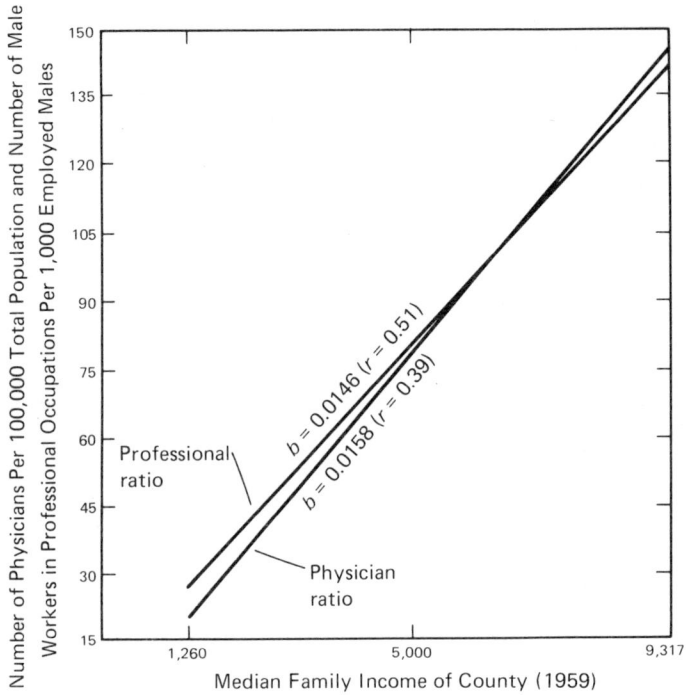

Y-axis label: Number of Physicians Per 100,000 Total Population and Number of Male Workers in Professional Occupations Per 1,000 Employed Males

Curve labels: $b = 0.0146$ ($r = 0.51$); $b = 0.0158$ ($r = 0.39$); Professional ratio; Physician ratio

X-axis label: Median Family Income of County (1959)

Figure 3-1. Regression of Physician and Professional Ratios on Median Family Income

Findings for the relationship between the two ratios and the urban index are generally similar, although the regression coefficient is higher for the physician ratio (0.891 versus 0.598). As noted, however, the correlations are virtually identical (0.44 and 0.46).

---

by differences in variation in the professional and physician ratios. Variation in the professional ratio is about 100 times greater than variation in the physician ratio; the average percentage of the male labor force in professional and technical occupations (that is, the number of professionals per 100 labor force), is 106 times the number of physicians per 100 total population (6.8 versus 0.064). One way to standardize the results from the regression analysis would be to multiply the results of the regression analysis for the physician ratio by 106. The same approximate effect is achieved by using 100,000 for the denominator in the physician ratio and 1,000 for the denominator in the professional ratio. We choose to report results as in Figure 3-1 so that a meaningful interpretation of the regression analysis can be given (that is, the number of physicians or professionals that can be expected on the average for a certain income level). (The use of standardized regression coefficients [Beta weights] would be useless in this case, since in the two variable case the standardized regression coefficient has the same value as the correlation coefficient.) There is no such problem for the correlation coefficients.

The common pattern can be seen another way. If the two ratios are influenced by community economic and urban characteristics the same way, the regression coefficients between indices of community structure and the two ratios should be related. For example, variation in the effect of community wealth on the professional ratio should be correlated with variation in the effect of community wealth on the physician ratio. Counties are divided into the nine regional divisions of the United States and regression coefficients between the two manpower ratios and median family income are computed for counties within each region. For example, the regression coefficients for the county physician and professional ratios on median family income are 9.8 and 9.5 respectively for the 470 counties in the West South Central region. We would expect that in regions where community wealth exerts a strong effect on the professional ratio we would find a strong effect on the physician ratio; that is, a correlation between the regression coefficients for the two ratios would be expected. The relationship can be seen in Figure 3-2; the tendency for the two coefficients to vary together is clear ($r = 0.57$).[j] It is also clear that were it not for the West North Central region (WNC), which has an unusually low regression coefficient for the professional ratio on median family income, the plots for the regions fit a straight line rather closely. This can be seen by the r of 0.88, which obtains when the West North Central region is eliminated from the analysis. The Spearman rank correlation is 0.67 for all nine regions and is 0.88 when the West North Central region is eliminated.

Independence of measures. The question of independence between the professional ratio and county income was discussed above. Comparing regression lines for the physician and professional ratios, as in Figure 3-1 and 3-2, also raises questions about the independence of measures. First, since physicians are included in the "professional and technical" category, the professional and physician ratios are not completely independent of each other. Consequently, the similarity of the two regression lines might be interpreted as a "part-whole" phenomenon. Of course, this is what the framework stipulates. The question arises, however, as to whether the results are due to a statistical artifact because the two ratios are not independent measures. That is, the professional ratio may vary with the physician ratio simply because physicians are included in the number of professional and technical workers. The seriousness of the problem is reduced considerably because the two ratios have different denominators. More important, according to the U.S. Census (which includes all federal as well as research, administrative, and faculty physicians in the enumeration), the total number of physicians constitutes only a small proportion (3.1%) of the total

[j]Regions are identified in Figure 3-2 according to initials: New England (NE), Middle Atlantic (MA), East North Central (ENC), West North Central (WNC), South Atlantic (SA), East South Central (ESC), West South Central (WSC), Rocky Mountain (RM), and Pacific Coast (PC).

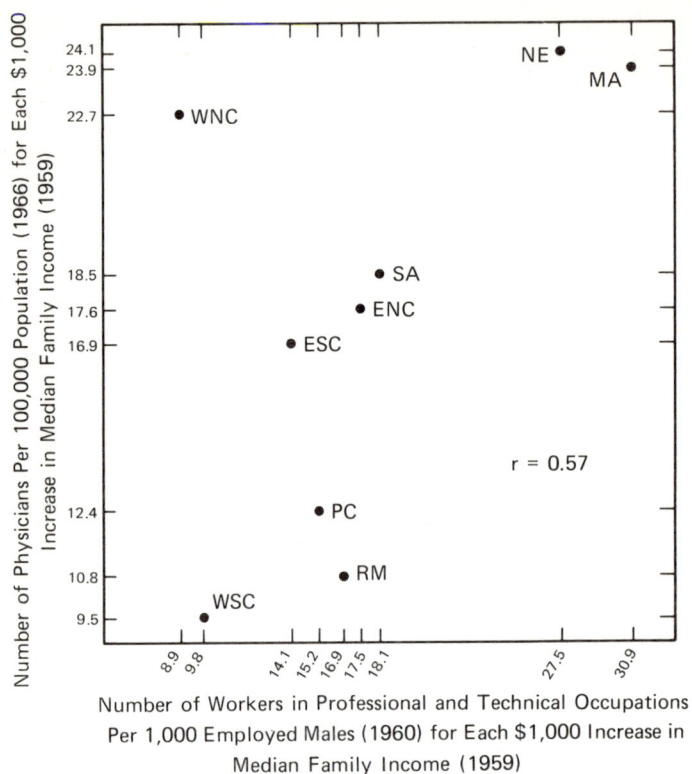

Figure 3-2. Plot of Regression Coefficients of Physician and Professional Ratios on County Median Family Income by Region

workers in the professional and technical category. In 1960 there were 230,307 physicians in comparison to 7,324,906 persons classified in professional and technical occupations (U.S. Bureau of the Census 1963a, pp. 1-2). Since our ratio includes only active nonfederal physicians in patient care, the actual percentage is even lower. Consequently, variation between counties in the professional ratio is at most only slightly mathematically determined by variation in the number of physicians.

A second issue concerns the lack of independence between the ratios and the measure of county income. Physicians and professional persons contribute to community wealth as reflected in the index of median family income. To some degree, therefore, both ratios are being regressed on themselves. The problem is more serious for the professional category, since it includes approximately 10 percent of the labor force (see page 40). Given the measurement of community wealth, there is no way to solve this particular problem. The matter is of no particular significance for physicians, since they constitute only a small proportion (less than 0.3 percent) of the total labor force (230,307 out of 68,001,553; U. S. Bureau of the Census 1963a, pp. 1-2). In addition, there are differences between types of physicians, which are examined in Chapter 7. If the results were due to an artifact of measurement, differences between types of physicians would not be expected.

At this point the problem may be pursued further by comparing the distribution of physicians and registered nurses. Since neither of these groups contribute very much to overall county wealth, it is not likely that the results will reflect a lack of independence between measures of county wealth and the manpower ratios for the two occupations. Ratios for the two groups are obtained for the 95 Tennessee counties. The number of physicians and nurses by county are obtained for the year 1962 from Maryland Y. Pennell and Kathryn I. Baker (1965), which gives the total number of federal (excluding military) and nonfederal physicians and the number of active nurses for each county. The population figures used to compute the ratios are for 1960 (U.S. Bureau of the Census 1962). The regression coefficients for the number of registered nurses and number of physicians per 100,000 on the 1959 median family income of counties are 0.0752 for nurses and 0.0413 for physicians (corresponding correlation coefficients are 0.76 and 0.70). If anything, the proportional effect of county wealth on the two ratios is somewhat greater for nurses; the tendency for wealthier counties to have higher ratios of health-care manpower is obviously not confined to physicians.

Therefore, similar relationships for the distribution of physicians and other professional personnel appear indeed to be the result of a general pattern and not an artifact of measurement.[k] The pattern is one in which communities with economic advantages tend to have advantages in other respects. Communities with a shortage of physicians tend also to have a shortage of other technically skilled and professionally trained persons. It is not just that physicians are specifically attracted to wealthier and more urban communities but that persons in professional and technical occupations in general are attracted to these communities. The locus of the problem is viewed with reference to the general pattern and in terms of community rather than the motives of physicians.

Evidence from studies of individual communities. The results and interpretation are also consistent with the descriptions provided by studies of individual small and medium communities in which economic problems are quite serious. (See Lyford 1962; Martindale and Hanson 1969; and West

---

[k]In addition, results for other health-care occupations in which the problem of independence of measurement does not exist are consistent with this conclusion. The results are presented in Chapter 13.

1945.) For example, Joseph Lyford, in a study of an economically depressed community, Vandalia, found that citizens were anxious about the "scarcity of jobs, lack of town leadership, the shortage of good housing, and the growing problems of the school system" (e.g., it was difficult to retain good teachers) (Lyford 1962, pp. 44-45). He was also told by a town lawyer:

> We have trouble keeping doctors. . . . There are four small towns in this county that have to go out and subsidize doctors to get decent medical attention to their people (Lyford 1962, p. 62).

The problem, however, is not limited to doctors (or to teachers).

> This is true of the bar, too. Our bar association has shrunk by 20 or 30 percent. Maybe we'll have to subsidize lawyers. This is serious not just because we need lawyers, but if you don't have lawyers where are you going to get the people who have always been most active in civic affairs and politics? (Lyford 1962, pp. 62-63.)

Vandalia, and the many other communities with a shortage of physicians, does not just have a problem of too few physicians. It has a shortage of persons in the professions in general, and it is a community in economic decline in which the survival of some of its basic social institutions is threatened. "The problem at the root of all the others is the economic decline of the entire county," indeed, a community that "is beset by the . . . desperate problem of how to hold on to what it has in order to survive" (Lyford, 1962, pp. 44, 218). And it is clear from Don Martindale and R. Galen Hanson's description of a similar community, Benson, that the declining economy of the local community and its weakened social institutions are related to forces in the broader society (Martindale and Hanson 1969, esp. pp. 81-111).

Of course, many communities which face serious physician shortages may not be in situations as dire as Vandalia and Benson — but some may be threatened even more. The fact is, however, that counties with general economic problems, at least as indicated by the low income of most of its families, do tend to have a shortage of physicians. The shortage is only one aspect of a more general problem. That problem and the forces that cause it are not apt to be seen if the maldistribution of physicians is viewed solely in terms of the motives physicians have for locating in some communities rather than others. Such interpretations need to be complemented with frameworks that explain why communities are as they are.

Changes in the Distribution of Physicians

A second implication of the framework that is pursued here concerns changes in the maldistribution of physicians. The framework indicates one of two alternative conclusions. The first is that since community wealth, size-density, and occupational-service sector are interdependent—with an increase in one leading to an increase in the other, an increase in community inequalities in physician manpower would be expected because physicians are part of the local occupational-service sector. A problem, however, is that the relationships among the three variables are far from perfect, so that other factors may intervene that prevent the rich communities from improving their position relative to the poor. For example, poor communities may provide free utilities, promise low taxes, and make other inducements that make an otherwise unattractive community attractive to thriving industries. In addition, as the occupational skill level of a community increases and attracts newer and higher paying industry, the older poorer paying industries must find some place to locate. As Wilbur Thompson's above quote (see pp. 42-43) suggests, they may locate in communities that are low on the economic scale of differences between communities. In this instance, both the wealthy and poor communities gain something. The second alternative outcome, then, would be the preservation of the existing differences, not the enhancement of the advantages of one in comparison to the other. Since the distribution of physicians is part of this broader pattern, no change in community inequalities would be expected. In the absence of a better theory of industry location and the interrelationship between industry and economy, size-density, and occupational skill mix, and the availability of more and better data than now exist, all that can be said is that inequalities between communities in physician manpower would be expected either to increase or remain stable over time. A decrease would not be expected.

Evidence lends support to this view. A study for the period 1923 to 1938 suggests that physicians concentrate increasingly in the wealthier more populous counties over time. Joseph W. Mountin, Elliott H. Pennell, and Virginia Nicolay divide United States counties into 11 groups, based on average per capita effective buying income in 1940. They then give the 1923 and 1938 physician-to-population ratio for each of the 11 county aggregates. Their results show that for the lowest income group, physicians per 100,000 decreased by 52 percent in this 18-year period. Moreover, the level of decrease-increase is systematically associated with the income class of the group of counties. All groups decreased except the highest income group; based on the figures reported, the percentage of decrease-increase (with a negative sign indicating a decrease) from the lowest income group to the highest are as follows: -52%; -49%; -47%; -32%; -29%; -12%; -18%; -14%; -8%; and +8%. (Mountin, Pennell, and Nicolay 1942c, p. 1947.) Note that the overall increase in population was also associated with income class, though less systematically than the physician ratio. (The increase was from 6 to 9% for the lowest seven groups on income, to 15%, 21%, and 22% increases for the top three on income.) (Mountin, Pennell, and Nicolay 1942c, p. 1947.) In comparing the ratios for the highest and lowest income groups, in 1923 there were 2.2 times as many physicians per 100,000 in the highest income group as in the lowest income group; by 1938 the highest income group had 3.3 times as many physicians per 100,000 as the lowest income group. The authors conclude, therefore, that "the growing tendency for physicians to select wealthy and populous counties for their practice becomes more pronounced with each succeeding year" (1942c, p. 1947).

More recent evidence suggests the trend has continued. The number of counties which had no physician is available for several years since 1950. Based on census figures reported by Maryland Y. Pennell and Marion E. Altenderfer (1954, pp. 56-172), there were 64 counties in 1950 in which no physician was in the employed labor force. According to reports by the American Medical Association, based on their annual questionnaire, there were 72 counties that had no active nonfederal physician in 1959 (Stewart and Pennell 1960, pp. 41-89), while in 1963 there were 98 counties that had no active nonfederal physician with the figure growing to 126 by 1968 (Haug et al. 1970, p. 23). For 1971 the AMA reported 131 counties without an active federal or nonfederal physician in patient care (Roback 1972, p. 12). Although the exact definition of physician varies somewhat in the different sources (census and AMA) and from time to time in the same source, the trend is clear: There were more counties with zero physician manpower in 1971 than in 1950.

Systematic analysis of all United States counties is difficult because of the nature of the available data. Results reported in the previous chapter were for nonfederal practicing physicians primarily engaged in patient care for the year 1966. Figures for this category of physicians are not available by county prior to 1963 (Theodore and Sutter 1966). Obviously a comparison of figures for 1963 and 1966 is of no value, since three years is much too short a period for physicians to be redistributed among counties to any significant degree. However, data are available for the number of physicians by county based on United States Census figures for 1950, which includes federal (excluding military) and nonfederal physicians, as well as other physicians not primarily engaged in patient care (such as administrative, research, and faculty physicians, as well as possibly some inactives); these data are reported by Pennell and Altenderfer (1954). Data are also available for all nonfederal physicians from the American Medical Association publication for 1966 (Theodore, Sutter, and Jokiel 1967). Although these data are not as useful for our purposes as data for nonfederal physicians primarily engaged in patient care, they will at least allow some tentative conclusions as to changes in the distribution of physicians from 1950 to 1966.

Given the probable tendency for physicians to remain in the county in which they establish their first practice,[1] as well as the probability that changes

---

[1]Although some research shows that many physicians do leave their place of initial practice (Benham, Maurizi, and Reder 1968; Mountin, Pennel, and Brockett 1945), there are strong "impediments to mobility" (Benham, Maurizi, and Reder 1968, p. 337) and some believe that "once a physician establishes a practice [in a community] . . . he is unlikely to move" (Bible 1970, p. 4; see also Steele and Rimlinger 1965, p. 188).

over a short space of 16 years in the proportion of new physicians who begin practice in different types of counties (e.g., rural versus urban) are quite small, very little change in the proportional distribution among United States counties would be expected in 16 years. Indeed, the correlation between the physicians per 100,000 county population in 1950 and 1966 is 0.76, indicating that high (low) ratio counties in 1950 were high (low) ratio counties in 1966. The correlation is not perfect, however, so that some change did occur. Nevertheless, given the magnitude of the correlation it is clear that the physician ratio of 1966 is in large part due to the physician ratio in 1950. Consequently, it will be necessary to control for this factor when investigating the effects of county economic and urban characteristics on changes in community physician manpower between 1950 and 1966.

To do this, the results for partial correlations and regressions are given between the physician ratio for 1966 and each of the two variables, county wealth and percent urban residents for 1960,[m] with the physician ratio for 1950 controlled. The partial correlations for community wealth and urban are extremely low, 0.03 for income and 0.12 for size-density. This means that county increases in physician manpower were only slightly related to community wealth and size-density. Partial regression coefficients indicate that a difference of $1,000 median family income in 1960 was worth, on the average, about 0.7 more physicians per 100,000 in 1966 than in 1950; and a difference of 1 percent in percentage of county residents living in urban areas was worth approximately 0.15 more physicians per 100,000 population in 1966 over 1950.[n] The change that did occur was slightly positively correlated with the economic and urban characteristics of communities.

A final observation is in order. Results reported in the previous chapter for the class of 1960 indicated that level of county income and percentage of urban residents interact in their effects on the physician ratio. Specifically, the positive effects of county income on the ratio are strongest for the least urban counties and are actually negative for the most urban counties; likewise, the positive effects of urban level are greatest for the poorest counties and negative for the wealthiest counties. These patterns and their relationship to the

---

[m]As was noted, figures for annual median family income of county are for 1959 rather than 1960.

[n]Zero-order correlations for the relationships between median family income (1959) and the 1950 and 1966 physician ratios are 0.48 and 0.38, and corresponding correlations for percentage of residents living in urban areas (1960) are 0.49 and 0.44. Standard deviations are 1,309 for median family income, 27.83 for percentage of urban residents, and 50.1 and 63.2 for the 1950 and 1966 physician manpower ratios respectively. Hence, regression coefficients for 1950 and 1966 physician ratios regressed on 1959 median family income are 0.0184 and 0.0183; for 1950 and 1966 physician ratios regressed on percentage of urban residents (1960) are 0.0084 and 0.0088; and the regression of 1966 physician ratio on 1950 physician ratio is 0.96. Sources of data: Pennell and Altenderfer (1954), U.S. Bureau of the Census (1952-1953; 1967), and Theodore, Sutter, and Jokiel (1967).

framework will be outlined in Chapter 6, at which time the role of suburbanization is discussed both with respect to the framework and the distribution of
physicians.

Conclusion

The physicians ratio of a county may be viewed as a property of the county
and as causally interrelated with other properties of the county. Causal statements may be made from this perspective without viewing the motives, values,
and attitudes of physicians as the primary causal factors. This is not to say that
this perspective is inconsistent with one that focuses on individual characteristics.
Rather, the two should be viewed as complementary. Certainly motives, values,
and attitudes are important factors in the location decisions of individual physicians. But insofar as they are involved in the maldistribution phenomenon, they
are probably not much different from those that characterize other professionally
and technically trained groups. More important, they themselves are only factors which influence how *individuals* respond to differences between communities;
they do not provide a framework for understanding the community differences
themselves. Although there is very little theory and empirical data to provide a
guide in the development of such a framework, the outline of a framework has
been presented. The framework is consistent with the findings in the previous
chapter for county income and urbanization, as well as results presented in this
chapter comparing the distribution of physicians with other professional groups
and the distribution of physicians at different points in time. It will provide a
theoretical orientation for the interpretation of the relationship between the
physician ratio and other variables that have been reported to be (or are commonly believed to be) related to the maldistribution of physicians. These
variables include community background, suburbanization, specialization, hospital facilities, and medical school policy. The framework also provides a guide
for the assessment of several policy programs and for the development of a
strategy to deal with the problem.

4

Community Production and Recruitment of Physicians

Thus far concern has been entirely with the place where physicians practice and, hence, on characteristics that serve communities in recruiting physicians. It would be expected, however, that these same characteristics also contribute to the production of physicians. The issue is important because it is possible that physicians tend to practice in the same or similar communities to those in which they were reared. One study, for example, reports that almost one half of the physicians who practice in small towns (less than 2,500) were reared in small towns (Bible 1970). Consequently, an examination of the community backgrounds of physicians is pertinent.

The chapter is divided into two parts. The first section outlines what the theoretical framework of the previous chapter stipulates in the way of community differences in the production of physicians, and findings for the class of 1960 are examined in light of those predictions. The second investigates the relationship between physicians' communities of origin and communities of practice.

Production of Physicians

There are several reasons for expecting wealthy urban counties to produce a disproportionate number of physicians. Such counties have a higher proportion of families with the economic ability to send their children to college and medical school. Also, wealthier more urban communities provide better elementary and secondary education for their children to attend, thus orienting and preparing them for higher education, and, subsequently, for professional careers such as medicine. Documentaries have been made of education in economically depressed rural and semirural communities, and the comparatively inferior quality of the education provided in such communities is widely believed. Several studies of small communities are consistent with this belief. (Lyford 1962; Martindale and Hanson 1969; West 1945.) The problem of attracting good teachers is difficult, and the good teachers are apt to leave. "The new teachers who come to Vandalia are usually bad risks [since they are apt to leave], because there are higher salaries elsewhere for them once they get experience . . . ." (Lyford 1962, p. 91). It may not be just a problem of economics and low teacher salaries; community attitudes which characterize such communities may inhibit the development of better educational systems. "The hostility to 'new

55

ideas' and to 'higher education' and the stressing in churches of the 'sins of the cities' are devices by which, whatever their other functions, parents strive to keep their children in Plainville, and effectively restrict their success when they leave" (West 1945, p. 220). Parents of such communities may be pulled between wanting their children to remain in the community and with providing them with good educations at the risk that they will leave. About one such community, Don Martindale and R. Galen Hanson state: "Because Benson on its own cannot assimilate all of its own children [occupational opportunities are too limited], Bensonites face the prospect that some of their offspring must make their way in the wider world. Benson's parents must either prepare their offspring for the metropolitan world or decrease their children's changes for success outside Benson. However, this very preparation for life outside may itself encourage the children to leave. In their view of education, Bensonites could be expected to be ambivalent. The whole sphere of socialization is subject to conflicting pulls." (Martindale and Hanson 1969, p. 60.) As a result many children may not be adequately prepared to pursue educations that lead to employment in occupations which require high level technical and professional skills, such as physicians.

In addition, wealthier more urban communities may produce more physicians simply because they recruit more. Individuals growing up in these communities are more apt to see wealthy and successful persons, as judged by general standards of society, because their communities have higher proportions of workers in professional occupations, including physicians. Such an environment encourages high educational and occupational aspirations among youth. In communities with high physician-to-population ratios, there are more physicians available in the community and neighborhood to advise youngsters on medical careers and to function as role models for them to follow. This is especially true with respect to the occupations of fathers; sons are apt to pursue the careers followed by their fathers than most other types of careers, especially if the father's career was in a higher status occupation (Blau and Duncan 1966, p. 28). For example, in the class of 1960, 321 had fathers who were physicians and another 19 had fathers in "other medical" occupations (veterinarians, osteopaths). This is 16.5 percent of 2,054 individuals whose fathers' occupations were reported. Another 20 were dentists, for a total percentage of approximately 17.5 percent in the high status medical and quasi-medical occupations. These occupations constitute less than 1 percent of the labor force.

In summary, children reared in affluent urban communities rather than poor rural areas are more apt to be aware of more occupational opportunities. They also attend higher quality educational institutions, and are encouraged to adopt high educational and occupational aspirations. Youngsters growing up in such an environment are more apt to be exposed to a community culture and to institutions that prepare them for, orient them toward, and motivate and support them in the pursuit of higher education and professional careers. Wealthier

urban counties more than poor, rural counties have the local institutions to produce, as well as to attract, physician manpower.

Data from the AAMC Longitudinal study will permit a test of this hypothesis. The analysis will parallel part of that in Chapter 2, which was in terms of the
number of physicians in 1972 per unit of population for 1970. The same procedure is used here except that the ratio is for the percentage of physicians in
the class of 1960 who originated from counties of designated income and urban
characteristics to the percentage of the population living in those counties in
1950 (the last census year prior to entering medical school). This gives a physician production ratio.

In the follow-up questionnaire of 1972, physicians were asked to give the
names of their places of birth. From this it was possible in 2,363 cases to determine the physicians' counties of birth, just as was done for counties of practice.
The income and urban characteristics of the counties was then obtained from
the U.S. Census in each case.[a] Since county differences in the production of
physicians are to be compared with differences in the recruitment of physicians
in the next section, it would be desirable to have measures of county income
and urbanization that are standardized with respect to the two points in time—
the time just prior to entering medical school, 1956, and the year in which the
follow-up questionnaire obtained the physician's county of practice, 1972.
In most instances the absolute income of a county and the percentage of urban
residents in 1956 are probably higher than the income and urban levels for the
same county in 1972. Consequently, the number of counties in the income
range of, say less than $3,000 median annual family income, will be smaller
in 1956 than in 1972. For this reason alone the number of physicians practicing in counties with less than $3,000 annual family income in terms of 1972
dollars will be smaller than the number of physicians who are classified as originating from counties in this income level based on 1956 dollars. In order to use
a common standard for comparing counties of origin and of practice, county
income and percent of urban residents for both origin and practice are for 1959

---

[a]While it would have been desirable to know the county in which the individual was
living just prior to medical school, such information is not available. It is probable, however,
that for many physicians the county of birth is the county in which they spent a large portion of their lives prior to medical school. Still, considering the high rate of mobility in the
United States, and the fact that these physicicans grew up during the years of World War II,
when some fathers were in the armed services, the percentage for whom the county of birth
is different from the county of residence just prior to medical school might be substantial.
Phillip Held (1973) has examined this problem with reference to states and regions and
concluded that this may indeed by the case for states and regions. Since the net migration
of individuals from time of birth to time of entering medical school probably favors movement from low-income and rural counties to high-income and urban counties, the percentage
of physicians who were actually living in low-income, rural counties just prior to medical
school may be lower than the analysis will show. Consequently, results may understate the
strength of the positive relationship between income-urbanization of communities and rate
of physician production.

and 1960, which are the measures used in the analysis in Chapter 2 for county
of practice. Since 1959-1960 falls between the time of entering medical school
and the county of practice in 1972, for neither the county of origin nor county
of practice will the income and urban measures be precisely accurate. It does
provide a common standard and this is what is needed.

It was observed in Chapter 2 that based on the physicians' counties of practice, the correlation between county income and the urban index is 0.45 for
physicians in the AAMC Longitudinal Study. Identical analysis was conducted
for the income and urban values for counties of origin. The product-moment
correlation is 0.59, which means that physicians who come from high income
counties tended also to come from the more urbanized counties. Table 4-1
gives the ratio of the percentage of physicians in counties, cross classified by
income and percent urban residents, to the percentage of the total population
living in those counties in 1950. As in Table 2-2, since the income and urban
levels of county of origin are correlated, it is difficult to make points of separation on both variables so that all income-urban combinations are represented,
or in which the percentages of physicians and total population are large enough
to permit reliable comparisons. The correlation is not so high as to preclude
meaningful analysis, however. Table 4-1 presents two sets of comparisons.
(Table 4-1 is based on 2,361 cases rather than 2,363 because the census does not
report the income for county of origin for two physicians.)

First, the separate effects of county income and urban level on the physician
production ratio may be seen from examining the column and row totals. The
column totals reveal that the ratio increases from counties with lower proportions
of urban residents to counties with higher proportions. Whereas counties with
fewer than 40.0 percent urban residents produced 13.08 percent of the physician
graduates, they had 20.96 percent of total 1950 physician population; consequently, they produced only 62 percent of their proportionate share. In comparison, counties with at least 90.0 percent urban residents produced 46.67 percent of the physicians but had only 33.01 percent of the total population;
consequently, they produced 141 percent of their proportionate share. A similar
trend is indicated for income, except that the ratio for the highest income
category is unusually low. In general, then, wealthier and more urban counties
are not only more apt to attract physicians; they are more apt to produce physicians as well.

A second form of analysis may be made of Table 4-1 by comparing the
ratios within rows and columns. This permits an assessment of the joint effects
of income and percent urban and the effect of each with the effects of the other
held constant. On balance, the effects of urban appear to be stronger than the
effects of income. Within all four columns, the physician ratio tends to increase
as the percentage of urban residents increases. Comparisions across rows for
income yields less consistent results. There is some indication that the ratio increases as income increases in counties with lower proportions of urban residents

Table 4-1
Ratio of Physician Percentage to Percentage of Population by County Income and Percent Urban Residents for Physician County of Origin—Class of 1960 (N = 2,361)

Percent Urban Residents (1960)	Median Family Income (1959)				
	Less Than $5,000	$5,000-$5,999	$6,000-$6,999	$7,000 and Above	Totals
90.0-100.0%	1.98[a] (2.14:1.08)[b]	1.67 (15.26:9.13)	1.52 (19.80:13.02)	0.97 (9.47:9.78)	1.41 (46.67:33.01)
80.0-89.9%	1.78[a] (3.08:1.73)	0.77 (3.00:3.90)	1.18 (5.83:4.96)	0.60 (2.06:3.44)	1.00 (13.97:14.03)
60.0-79.9%	0.77 (3.22:4.19)	0.97 (7.03:7.46)	1.06 (4.59:4.34)	0.62[a] (0.47:0.76)	0.93 (15.31:16.54)
40.0-59.9%	0.69 (5.23:7.53)	0.69 (4.16:6.07)	0.86[a] (1.59:1.85)	—	0.71 (10.98:15.45)
Less than 40.0%	0.55 (9.78:17.89)	0.74 (2.01:2.73)	3.79[a] (1.29:0.34)	—	0.62 (13.08:20.96)
Totals	0.72 (23.45:32.42)	1.08 (31.46:29.08)	1.35 (33.10:24.51)	0.86 (12.00:13.98)	1.00 (100.00:100.00)[c]

Sources: AAMC Longitudinal Study and U.S. Bureau of Census (1952-1953, 1967).
[a]Denotes low percentages for physician and total population.
[b]Figures in parenthesis are percentage of physician (by origin) : percentage of 1950 population.
[c]Percentages may add to more or less than 100 percent because of rounding error.

and decreases with income for counties with higher proportions. At the same
time, if we ignore the highest income category as well as the cells where the
percentages are low, the joint effects of income and urban level are clear: The
ratios in cells toward the upper right corner of the table are much higher than
those toward the lower left corner.

Findings are therefore consistent with the hypothesis based on the framework in the previous chapter. Counties with high income and a high proportion
of urban residents have institutions that produce a disproportionately large
number of physicians whereas the institutions of low income, rural communities produce a disproportionately small number. A number of factors are no
doubt involved. These include the ones discussed above, although other factors
may also be present. In addition, the exact processes may be different from
those that were posited. These questions aside, it is clear that community
differences in productivity rates are to be explained only in terms of community
characteristics. They are not adequately explained by characteristics of individuals, such as economic motivation. Of course, individuals from poor rural communities may differ in personality and motivational characteristics from individuals reared in wealthy urban communities, and these differences may be
important factors in whether a person goes to medical school and subsequently
becomes a physician. Even so, why and how different types of environments
produce different motivational orientations in individuals would need to be
explained. But in any case, the differences observed in Table 4-1 are between
different types of communities (that is, counties). Therefore, community
characteristics rather than individual characteristics are probably the causal
factors. Frameworks based on a theory of individual behavior are not only
inadequate for explaining why communities differ in the characteristics which
serve to attract physicians; they are inadequate for explaining the effect those
characteristics have in producing physicians.

As noted, there are a number of missing cases since county of origin is known
for only 2,363 of the original 2,821 students. Conclusions based on Table 4-1
would not likely be changed even if the missing cases were unevenly distributed
in counties of different income and urban levels. If the missing cases were disproportionately concentrated in low-income, rural counties, it would indicate
that such counties probably produce poorer students (more dropouts) as well as
fewer than their proportionate share of the graduates. If a disproportionate
number came from high-income counties, it would merely indicate that such
counties produce a higher proportion of unsuccessful as well as successful
students.

**Relationship Between Production and
Recruitment**

These results suggest that one reason higher income more urban counties get more than their proportionate share of physicians is because they produce more than their proportionate share. This assumes that physicians tend to practice in the types of communities in which they were reared. It is possible, however, that the tendency is not a strong one. Consequently, differences in the county production of physicians may have little if any causal significance for county differences in the supply of physicians. For county differences in the production of physicians to be a causal factor, there would have to be a relationship between the characteristics of physicians' counties of origin and their counties of practice.

Study of the relationship between counties of origin and practice is an analysis of the degree to which physicians move from one place to another. In viewing this general process authors have emphasized two specific processes: the "entry-exit" process and intercommunity migration. The entry-exit process refers to the number of new physician graduates who establish their initial practice in a community relative to the number who die and retire; when the latter exceeds the former, the ratio decreases. (This assumes of course that the total population does not change. It also assumes that physicians only terminate their practice in the community through death and retirement.) Second, community differences in the physician-population ratio may occur through in- and out-migration (intercommunity migration). If the total population does not change and if the entries and exits balance out, changes in the physician-to-population ratio is a function of the difference between in- and out-migrants. Different authors have focused on the entry-exit and the migration mechanisms as the crucial factors in differences between areas in physician manpower ratios. (See Benham, Maurizi, and Reder 1968; Mountin, Pennel, and Brockett 1945; Steele and Rimlinger 1967.)

A limitation of both views is that they do not indicate where physicians originally come from. Study of the entry-exit process only tells the number of physicians who establish their initial practice in a community over a period of time relative to the number who die or retire there during that period, and inter-community migration only indicates where physicians come from, and go, after having established their initial practice. Such data are adequate to establish the flow of physicians once they have graduated from medical school, and evidence does indicate that higher income counties have more entries relative to the number of exits than low income counties (Mountin, Pennel, and Brockett 1945) and that the movement of physicians from places with small populations to places of larger population is more frequent than the reverse process (Benham, Maurizi, and Reder, 1968; Mountin, Pennel, and Brockett 1945). Here, however, it is the flow of physicians from their place of residence prior to entering medical school in 1956 to their place of practice in 1972 that is being examined. Specifically, the effect of income and urban characteristics of physicians' counties of origin on where physicians subsequently practice is investigated. Results will be presented separately for county income and urban level.

Community Income, Production, and
Recruitment

Results for income are presented in cross tabular form in Table 4-2 for 2,285 physicians for whom the income both of county of origin and of practice are known. Before examining this table in detail, several observations are in order. If the correlation between income of counties of origin and counties of practice were perfect, physicians would be practicing in 1972 in counties that were identical in 1959 income to the counties in which they were reared. Counties of different income levels would get exactly the same number of physicians they produced. In this case, the correlation and regression coefficients between income for counties of origin and of practice would be 1.00.[b] In Table 4-2 all physicians would fall in the underlined diagonal cells, so that 100.0 percent of physicians from each income interval would be practicing in counties in that interval. Hence, the regression line would be located along the diagonal. Such a finding would seriously question the hypothesis that physicians tend to concentrate in higher income areas because of the greater economic (or other) opportunities offered by higher income areas. It would suggest quite a different hypothesis, namely, that physicians tend to locate in communities that permit the style of life to which they have become accustomed through socialization in their communities of origin.

If, however, community background had no influence on subsequent location decisions, the correlation and regression coefficients would be zero or near zero; where a physician came from would be irrelevant to where he subsequently practiced. In this case, the diagonal cells, which represent the percentage of physicians from counties of origin in each of the income intervals who also practice in counties in that interval, would have the same percentage as all physicians, given in the total column. More generally, the percentage distribution would be the same for all columns, and identical to the distribution for the totals column. Under this circumstance, the regression line would be horizontal and drawn at the point above and below where 50 percent of the cases fall, which is in the $6,000-$6,999 interval.

A third possibility is that the correlation is neither zero nor perfect. This would occur if location decisions are influenced both by community background and differences in economic and other opportunities offered by communities. In this case, the correlation and regression coefficients would be greater than 0.00 but less than 1.00 and the percentages in the diagonal cells of each column in Table 4-2 would be less than 100 percent but higher than the percentage in the totals column corresponding to the row of the diagonal cell. Results are

---

[b]Values of 1.00 for both product-moment correlation and regression coefficients are possible only when both variables in the relationship have the same metric. Since income for county of origin and of practice are for 1959, they have a common metric.

Table 4-2
Relationship Between Income of Physician's County of Origin and Income of Physician's County of Practice, in Percentages—Class of 1960

Income of County of Practice	Income of County of Origin[a]						
	Less Than $3,000	$3,000-$3,999	$4,000-$4,999	$5,000-$5,999	$6,000-$6,999	$7,000 and Over	Totals
$7,000 and over	4.2	9.7	13.4	24.3	20.5	46.3	22.6
$6,000-$6,999	14.6	20.8	27.1	27.8	49.9	25.6	33.6
$5,000-$5,999	25.0	31.2	29.1	37.4	20.9	21.0	28.0
$4,000-$4,999	29.2	18.8	25.3	8.5	7.4	5.7	11.5
$3,000-$3,999	12.5	14.9	3.8	1.3	1.2	1.4	3.0
Less than $3,000	14.6	4.5	1.4	0.7	0.1	0.0	1.4
D[b]	0.9507	0.9485	0.9100	0.8598	0.7917	0.8070	
N	96	154	292	719	743	281	

Sources: AAMC Longitudinal Study and U.S. Bureau of the Census (1967).

Note: County income for both county of origin and county of practice is for 1960.

[a]Column may not add to 100.0 percent because of rounding error.

[b]D adjusted for its maximum value (see text).

consistent with this. The product-moment correlation (*r*) between income of county of origin and of practice is 0.39 and the regression coefficient (*b*) is 0.352.^c And in each of the six income intervals, the percentage in the diagonal cell is substantially higher than the percentage in the total column (for example, 14.6% of physicians from counties with less than $3,000 income practice in these counties, in comparison to 1.4% for all physicians).

Table 4-2 also shows that the probability a physician will practice in a county in the same income range as the one in which he was reared increases almost continuously as the income level of the county increases—from 14.6 percent for the poorest counties to 46.3 percent for the wealthiest counties. This would seem to suggest that the influence of community of origin on location patterns increases as the income level of the community of origin increases. That is, the experience of growing up in a wealthy area apparently leads one to return to such an environment more than the experience of growing up in a poor area leads one to return to a poor area. This does not follow from the results, however. Comparisons of percentages within rows provide meaningful estimates of the influences of origin on practice location; one may say, for example, that the percentage of physicians from counties below $3,000 are about three times as likely as physicians from the $3,000-$3,999 range to locate in counties below $3,000 income (14.6% versus 4.5%—row 1, Table 4-2). Comparisons within columns are not meaningful. For example, although physicians from counties below $3,000 are twice as likely to locate in counties in the $4,000-$4,999 range as in counties below $3,000 (29.2% to 14.6%), this is partly because a much higher percentage of *all* physicians (totals column) locate in counties in the $4,000-$4,999 range (11.5% versus 1.4%). The probable reason for the distribution in the totals column is that higher income counties provide greater occupational opportunities for physicians, as well as more social and cultural opportunities for themselves and their families, as noted previously. The percentage in the diagonal, then, is a function of two things: the tendency to seek an environment similar to the one in which one was reared and the tendency to seek environments that provide the most in economic, social, and cultural opportunities. Therefore, the influence of origin alone is not reflected in the absolute cell percentage, but in the percentage of physicians who practice in counties similar to their counties of origin relative to the percentage of all physicians who practice in these counties. Consequently, the ratio of the percentage in each underlined diagonal cell to the total percentage is an index of how much more attractive counties of a certain income range are to physicians. Since 14.6 percent of physicians from the lowest income level practice in

---

^cThe *r* is statistically significant at the .00001 level. The correlation ratio (η) (with columns for less than $3,000, $3,000-$3,999, $4,000-$4,999, $5,000-$5,999, $6,000-$6,999, and $7,000 and over) is 0.38, which in is almost identical to the *r* of 0.39, thus indicating that the relationship is linear.

counties of this income range but only 1.4 percent of all physicians do so, the ratio is 10.4. This means that the poorest counties are over 10 times more attractive to physicians who grew up in these counties than they are to all physicians. Computations yield the following ratios for the diagonal cells for the other five income levels, from the lowest ($3,000-$3,999) to the highest ($7,000 and over): 4.97, 1.27, 1.34, 1.49, and 2.08[d] This would seem to suggest that the tendency for physicians to locate in counties similar in income to their counties of origin is strongest for physicians from the poorest counties. A difficulty in such a conclusion is that the results are partially an artifact of the small numbers who practice in low-income counties—31 and 68 in the two lowest intervals (which give percentages of 1.4 percent and 3.0 percent in the totals column). Consequently, small changes in the numbers in the diagonals of the first two columns would give much different results. For example, if 10 physicians in the diagonal of the first column practiced in higher categories, the ratio between the diagonal and the total would be 4.6 (4.2:0.9), less than half the current ratio of 10.4. Identical changes in the other columns would have a far less effect on the ratio.

The problem can be seen from a different perspective. Since 100 percent is the highest figure possible for the diagonal cell, the highest ratio possible between the percentage in the diagonal cell and the percentage in the appropriate row of the totals column is set by the percentage in the totals column. This means that the maximum value possible for the ratio decreases as the percentage in the totals column increases. Thus the maximum ratio possible for the diagonal cell in the first column is 71.4 (100% divided by 1.4%) whereas the maximum possible for the diagonal of the last column is only 4.42 (100% divided by 22.6%). Therefore, to some extent differences in the ratio between the percentage in the totals column and the internal columns may be artifacts of differences in the percentages in the totals column. In order to reduce the problem and make the percentages in the totals column more nearly equal, the bottom three rows and first three columns are combined, so that we have four columns (less than $5,000, $5,000-$5,999, $6,000-$6,999, and $7,000 and over). The column percentage for the lowest income category (less than $5,000) then becomes 15.9 (the sum of 1.4, 3.0, and 11.5). Of all physicians who originate from counties in this income range, 39.3 percent (213 of 542) subsequently practice in counties in this range, which gives a ratio of 2.47 (39.3%:15.9%). This is considerably lower than the ratios for the two poorest county groups in Table 4-2, but still considerably higher than 1.00. Thus the tendency for physicians to locate in counties similar in income to their counties of origin exists for physicians from

---

[d]The values here are subject to minor rounding errors. The precise method for obtaining the expected percentage for a cell is to multiply the corresponding percentages in the totals row and column and divide by 100%.

all origins (all ratios for the diagonal cells to the corresponding figure in the totals column are above 1.00).

This of course is indicated by the overall summary measures given by the correlation and regression coefficients. Since wealthier counties produce a disproportionately large share of physicians, the existence of a positive relationship assures that wealthier counties get more than their proportionate share of practicing physicians. In fact, the nature of the relationship is such that higher income counties get a larger proportionate share than they would get if a relationship did not exist. Discussion will make this clear.

The less than perfect correlation indicates that factors besides county of origin are involved in location patterns, such as the search for occupational, social, and cultural opportunities. Of course, the correlation of less than 1.00 might be due partially to sampling errors and errors of measurement rather than to the effects of community differences in opportunity. Results for another sample of physicians might show a much higher correlation and the magnitude of the correlation for the present sample might have been reduced because some individuals erroneously reported their county of birth and their county of practice in the study questionnaire; also, clerical errors may have occurred in the recording of income of counties of origin and practice from the census. But, if the less than perfect correlation were due to random errors of measurement, the percentages in the nondiagonal cells within each column would be about equal, that is, movement to poorer counties would be about the same as movement to richer counties. Analysis shows this is not the case. The distributions of physicians from counties with lower incomes (columns to the left of the diagonal) are more even than distributions for physicians from counties with higher incomes (columns to the right of the diagonal). For example, with the 14 physicians in the diagonal cell of the first column eliminated (14.6% of 96), the percentage distribution of the remaining 84 physicians in the other five cells is 14.3%, 33.3%, 28.6%, 16.7%, and 4.8%. This compares with the distribution of the 151 physicians in the last column with the 130 physicians (46.3% of 281) from the diagonal eliminated: 0.0%, 2.6%, 10.6%, 39.1%, and 47.7%. It is clear that physicians from the poorest income origins are more evenly distributed in counties above their origins than physicians from the wealthiest income origins are distributed in counties below their origins. Physicians from poorer origins are dispersed across county income levels to a greater extent than physicians from wealthier origins.

Therefore, comparison of columns in Table 4-2 indicates that the dispersal of physicians across income levels of counties of practice decreases from high-income to low-income counties of origin. A method is available for systematically comparing the dispersion-concentration within a column and is given by the following formula:[e]

---

[e]The method was first presented in Jack P. Gibbs and Walter T. Martin (1960).

$$D = 1 - \frac{\Sigma\,X^2}{(\Sigma\,X)^2} \quad,$$

where X is the percentage of persons in each row of each column. A low value indicates low concentration and high dispersion. If physicians in a column were concentrated in one row the result would be $1 - (1)(100^2) / (100)^2 = 0.0$. If, however, physicians were evenly distributed there would be 16.67 percent in each of the column cells, since there are six cells per column; in this case, the above formula would give the following result: $1 - (6)(16.67^2) / 100^2 = 0.8333$. Thus, for six rows, the maximum value of D is 0.8333.

A limitation of this measure is that when the rows vary the maximum values also vary; for example, if there were five rows the maximum value would be 0.8000 rather than 0.8333 $[1 - (5)(20.0^2)/(100^2)]$. Consequently, variation in the maximum value exists whenever there are empty cells, as in the highest income column in Table 4-2. This makes comparisons problematic since the standard of comparison is not uniform for all columns. The problem can be corrected, however, by dividing D by its maximum value (D_{max}), which is given by $1 - 1/N$, where N is the number of cells per column. The maximum value for D_{max} is 1.00 and the minimum is 0.0 regardless of the number of cells. Because one column in Table 4-2 has one empty cell, values for D/D_{max} are reported at the bottom of Table 4-1. Values almost continuously decrease from a high of 0.9507 for the lowest income counties to 0.8070 for the highest income counties. Since inspection shows that the pattern is for physicians to concentrate increasingly in high income counties as the income of county of origin increases, the decrease in D values from low-income to high-income counties of origin means that the dispersal of physicians from one income level to another systematically decreases as income level of community of origin increases. This means, in effect, that physicians from poorer counties are more evenly distributed than physicians from wealthier counties across counties of different income levels.[f]

To summarize, results in Table 4-2 reflect two processes: One is indicated by the relationship between income levels of community of origin and practice and is the process of physicians locating in communities that are similar (or the same) as the ones in which they were reared. Although the motivational roots of this tendency are not well understood, it probably involves the individual's desire to achieve a life-style similar to the one in which he was socialized. At the same time, newly graduated physicians may think they can establish an economically lucrative practice sooner in their home or similar communities than in other settings. The fact that a higher proportion of physicians from higher

---

[f]Examination of Table 4-2 shows this to be the case without the analysis based on D values. However, D provides a more systematic and summary form of analysis.

income, more urban areas practice in familiar settings may be due to the interaction of the desire for a familiar life-style with economic motivation. But regardless of motivation, the relationship is clear.

The other process is reflected in the D values along with the relationship
between incomes for county of origin and county of practice. Physicians from
low-income counties are more evenly distributed across all income levels than are
physicians from high-income counties. Consequently, the process of physicians
of all origins locating more in higher income areas counteracts the tendency of
physicians from low-income origins to locate in counties similar to their counties
of origin. As a result, low-income counties help to supply wealthier counties
with physician manpower.

Production, Recruitment, and Urbanization

The finding that the community production ratio of physicians is directly
related to the urban level of a community suggests that this may be a cause for
the relationship between community urban level and the practicing physician
ratio. To investigate this possibility, analysis for percentage of urban residents
is conducted identical to that for income in the previous section. The product-
moment correlation and regression coefficients are 0.28 and 0.221, thus supporting the hypothesis.[g] A migration matrix such as that for income in Table
4-2 was also constructed (see Table 1, Appendix C). In this case the matrix is
based on 10 distinctions—less than 10.0% ... 90.0-100.0%. The percentages in
the diagonal cells, given in order from counties of origin with the smallest to the
largest percentage of urban residents, are as follows: 3.8%, 3.7%, 9.2%, 8.3%,
15.7%, 18.8%, 19.7%, 25.0%, 35.3%, and 58.8%. Although each is considerably
less than the maximum of 100 percent, the ratio of each to the appropriate percentage in the total column is above 1.00 (see Table 1, Appendix C). This
means that the tendency to locate in the same county (or one that is similar in
level of urbanization) exists for physicians from the most rural origins as well
as for those from the most urban origins. Deviations from a perfect correlation
are due in large measure to the greater ability of more urban areas to attract
physicians. This is seen from the D values. Values by level of urbanization,
from counties of origin with less than 10.0 percent urban residents to those with
90.0 to 100.0 percent, are as follows: 0.9235, 0.9574, 0.9311, 0.9064, 0.9027,
0.8848, 0.9098, 0.8758, 0.8133, and 0.6768. Values almost continuously
decrease from the least urban to most urban counties[h] (see Table 1, Appendix

---

[g]The r is statistically significant at beyond the .00001 level; the correlation ratio (η)
is .30, with ten columns (less than 10.0% urban residents ... 90.0%–100.0% urban residents).
Source of data on percent urban residents is U.S. Bureau of the Census (1967).

[h]The Spearman-rank correlation between the rank of the D and the rank of urban level
for the ten intervals in Table C-1 of Appendix C is .89.

C). And since the overall tendency is for physicians to be attracted to the more urban counties, physicians from the less urban counties are more evenly dispersed across counties of different rural-urban levels than are physicians from more urban counties. The pattern is similar to that for county income.

Conclusion

Differences in community institutions, as these are determined by community differences in income and urban levels, are important determinants of the production of physicians. This is consistent with the theoretical framework in the previous chapter. Institutional differences between communities are shaped by macrosocial and macroeconomic events and processes that are external to physicians. The motivation to return to an environment like the one of origin may be an important factor in the distribution of physicians, but such motivation is itself the product of socialization processes and thus has its base in the social institutions of communities. These processes plus the overall greater attraction of higher income counties produce the paradox of low-income, rural counties producing less than their proportionate share of physicians but of helping to supply high-income, urban counties with physicians more than high-income, urban counties help to supply low-income, rural counties.

5

Community Consequences of the
Discrepancy in the Number of Physicians
Produced and Recruited

The nature of the relationships between income and urban levels of community of origin and community of practice have an important implication. They indicate that lower income, rural communities suffer a greater disadvantage than just a low supply of physicians. They also get fewer physicians than they produce. In this chapter the discrepancy in the number produced and recruited is investigated in more detail. Results are then examined with reference to a general pattern of migration from low-income, rural communities to high-income, urban communities.

County Income

Figure 5-1 distinguishes between seven income levels. The number of physicians produced (according to county of origin) and received (according to county of practice); each is then plotted on the midpoint of each income interval.[a] The two distributions are quite similar; the trend lines are approximately parallel. This is because the number of physicians produced and number recruited are both related to county wealth. But the trend lines are not perfectly parallel since they intersect.

The fact that the point of intersection is toward the middle of the income scale reveals that counties in the low end of the scale produce more physicians than they receive while those in the upper range produce fewer than they receive. Not only do richer counties get more than their proportionate share of physicians based on their share of the total population, as was seen in Chapter 2; they also get more than they actually produce, with the reverse being the case for poorer counties. Poor counties are drained of the physician talent they actually produce.

---

[a]A problem arises in establishing the midpoints for the extreme categories—less than $3,000 and $8,000 and over. The lowest and highest income counties are different for counties of origin and counties of practice. The poorest county in which a physician originated has $1,471 and the wealthiest $9,977. Corresponding figures for counties of practice are $1,877 and $9,551. The procedure for getting common midpoints is as follows. For the less than $3,000 category for county of origin, the range is $1,471 to $3,000, making the midpoint $2,236. The range for county of practice is $1,877 to $3,000, with a midpoint of $2,439. The midpoint in Figure 5-1 is the average of the two midpoints, which is $2,338. Using a similar procedure for the highest income interval ($8,000 and above), the midpoint is $8,883.

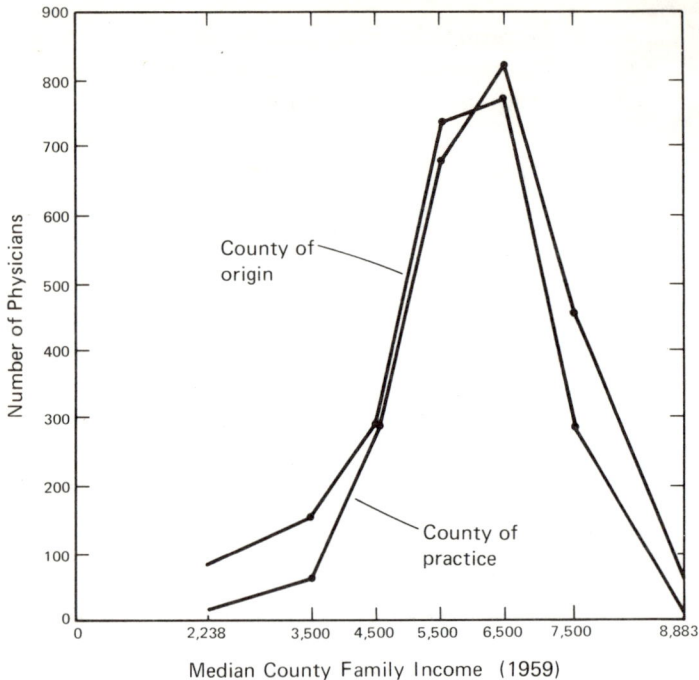

Figure 5-1. Plot of Physicians Produced (by County of Origin) and Received (by County of Practice) on Midpoint of Income for Seven Income Intervals

From one perspective, Figure 5-1 underestimates the actual extent of the discrepancy. This is so because the largest discrepancies occur at the extremes where there are fewer physicians. For example, counties with less than $3,000 median family income produced only 99 physicians and recruited 33, so that they produced exactly three times as many as they recruited, whereas counties with median family income of $8,000 and above produced only 18 but recruited 95, thus producing only 19 percent of the number they recruited. However, counties between $4,000 and $7,000 recruited about as many as they produced; for example, counties in the $5,000-$5,999 range recruited 671, which is 91 percent of the 741 they produced.

At the same time, Figure 5-1 may overestimate the actual discrepancies. This is so because the discrepancies are based on the absolute number of physicians originating and practicing in different types of counties and not the number relative to the population in the different types of counties. The absolute size of the population in most counties increased along with the total population from the time physicians entered medical school in 1956 to 1972. Therefore, although results unequivocally show discrepancies in the production and recruitment of physicians by county income level, discrepancies in terms of manpower *ratios* are not clear. Manpower ratios we recall are based on the number of physicians to the total population. Lower income counties may have lost population and higher income counties gained population from the time students entered medical school in 1956 to 1972. For example, whereas only 13.98 percent of the 1950 population were in counties that in 1959 had a median family income of at least $7,000, 18.54 percent of the 1970 population were in these counties (U.S. Bureau of the Census, 1952-1953; 1967; 1973a). Consequently, differences in the distributions for the production and recruitment of physicians may be the same as the differences in the distribution of the total population between 1956 and 1972. Analysis shows that this is not the case, however.

Since members of the 1960 class entered medical school in 1956 and most entered college in 1952, the population for 1950 is the denominator in computing the number of student physicians produced per 100,000 population. The population for 1970 is the denominator in computing the number of practicing physicians per 100,000 population. The resulting ratios will be referred to as the "production rate" and the "recruitment rate." Overall there was an increase in total population (excluding Alaska, District of Columbia, Hawaii, and Virginia), from 146,576,000 in 1950 to 196,738,000 for 1970 (U.S. Bureau of Census, 1973a). Since there were 2,514 physicians with known addresses in 1972, there were 1.72 entering medical students who subsequently graduated per 100,000 population in 1950 and 1.28 physicians in practice per 100,000 population in 1970. The ratio of 1.28 to 1.72 is 0.75. If the discrepancies as presented in Figure 5-1 are simply reflections of population change, with the higher income counties increasing their populations at a faster rate than the lower income counties, the ratios for counties in different income intervals should all be on the order of 0.75. Table 5-1 indicates that this is not the case.

First, note that the ratio between the overall recruitment rate and production rate is 0.76 rather than 0.75 (totals column). This stems from the fact that although there are 2,514 physicians with known addresses in the 1960 cohort, income of county of origin is known for only 2,361 and county of practice for only 2,418. Using these figures, the number of students per 100,000 population in 1950 is 1.61 and the number of physicians in 1972 per 100,000 population in 1970 is 1.23;[b] the ratio of 1.23 to 1.61 is 0.76. Comparison shows, however, that the ratio is much lower than this in the lowest income counties (0.37 and 0.41 for counties in the less than $3,000 and $3,000-$3,999 ranges) than in the highest income counties (1.03 for counties in the $7,000 income range). For

---

[b]Ratios are computed by dividing 2,361 by 146,671,280 and 2,418 by 196,730,000 and multipling each by 100,000.

Table 5-1
Physician Recruitment and Production Rates and Recruitment-Production Ratios, by County Income

	Median Family Income (1959)						
	Less Than $3,000	$3,000-$3,999	$4,000-$4,999	$5,000-$5,999	$6,000-$6,999	$7,000 and Above	Totals[a]
Recruitment Rate (RR)[b]	0.32	0.50	0.94	1.24	1.54	1.48	1.23
Production Rate (PR)[c]	0.86	1.22	1.29	1.73	2.14	1.43	1.61
Ratio of RR to PR	0.37	0.41	0.73	0.72	0.72	1.03	0.76

Sources: AAMC Longitudinal Study and U.S. Bureau of Census (1952; 1953; 1967; 1973a; 1973b).

[a] Totals for physicians: 2,418 for county of practice (for recruitment rate) and 2,361 for county of origin (for production rate). Totals for population: 196,730,000 for computing recruitment rate and 146,671,280 for computing production rate (see "County Income" this chapter for explanation).

[b] Number of physicians by county of practice per 100,000 population in 1970.

[c] Number of physicians by county of origin per 100,000 population in 1950.

counties between the extremes, the ratios are approximately the same as for the total population. This means, therefore, that the rate of out-migration for the lowest income counties by persons who became physicians was greater than the out-migration of the total population from these areas. (This assumes that differences in the population for counties of different income levels were not due substantially to differences in the birth rate.) Therefore, discrepancies in Figure 5-1 reflect real differences; even when size of population is standardized, lower income counties got fewer physicians than they produced whereas higher income counties got more than they produced.

County Urban Index

In Figure 5-2 trend lines connect the number of physicians produced and number recruited plotted against the midpoint of urban values for each of the 10 county groups stratified according to percent of residents living in urban areas.[c] It is clear that the distributions for the urban index differ from those for income, with both the number produced and recruited increasing continuously as percent urban residents increases. As with the distributions for income, however, the line for county of practice is below that for county of origin at the lower end of the urban scale but above it toward the upper end, except for counties with the highest urban values. The intersection of lines toward the middle of the scale reveals that the more rural counties get fewer physicians than they produce with the reverse situation obtaining for the more urban counties; rural counties help supply urban areas with physicians.

Note, however, that there was also a shift in the total population from rural areas to urban areas between the time this cohort of physicians entered college and 1972. For example, 36.45 percent of the population lived in counties with fewer than 60.0 percent urban residents in 1950 in comparison to 31.19 percent in 1970.[d] Hence, the movement of rural-reared physicians to urban counties may have been no greater than the overall movement in the population. Results in Table 5-2, which is identical to Table 5-1 except that counties are stratified according to percent of urban residents, rather than annual median family income, indicate otherwise. Again, the ratio of the number of physician students per 100,000 persons in the 1950 population to the number of physicians per 100,000 persons in the 1970 population is given; after standardizing for

---

[c]There is no problem of establishing common midpoints for counties of origin and of practice on the urban index for the lowest and higher intervals (below 10.0% and 90.0% and above), since the range of urban values for both counties of origin and practice is 0.0 percent to 100.0 percent.

[d]Source of data: U.S. Bureau of the Census (1952-1953; 1967; 1973a). However, the proportion living in the most urban counties remained about the same (see below).

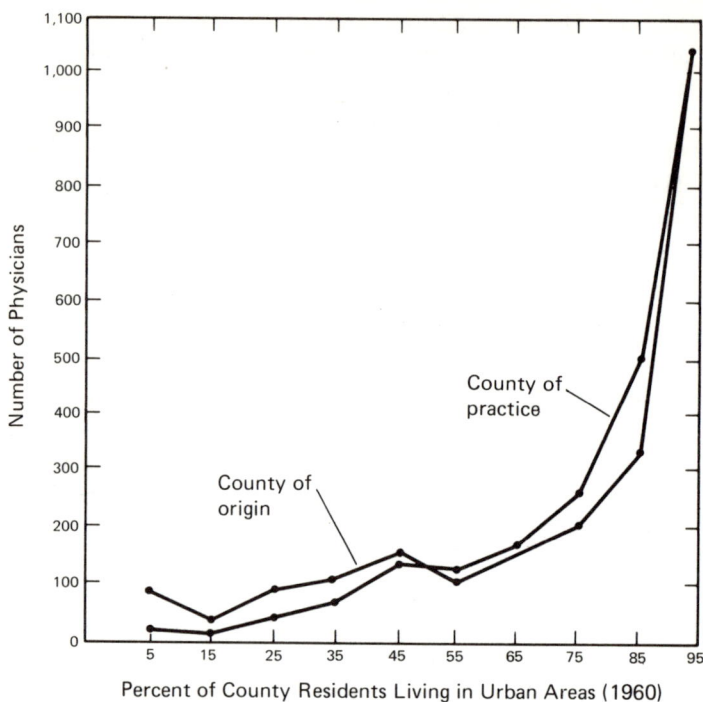

Figure 5-2. Plot of Physicians Produced (by County of Origin) and Received (by County of Practice) on Midpoint of County Average Percent of Urban Residents for Ten Urban Intervals—Class of 1960

population, if the ratio for a county group is in excess of 0.76, that group re-cruited a higher proportion of the physicians produced than county groups below 0.76. As Table 5-2 reveals, the recruitment-production ratio tends to increase as the percentage of urban residents increases. Unlike for income, the relationship is not continuous since the figure for the most urbanized group is lower than all other groups except those with fewer than 50.0 percent urban residents. Since the proportion of the total population living in the most urban group of counties remained almost constant from 1950 to 1970 (33.0 percent to 33.44 percent),[e] the lower recruitment-production ratio for the most urban counties stems from a smaller proportion of physicians practicing in those counties than the propor-tion who were reared there. Therefore, the pattern of discrepancies in the num-ber recruited and produced in Figure 5-2—the pattern for the most rural counties

---

[e]Source of data: U.S. Bureau of the Census (1952-1953; 1967; 1973a).

Table 5-2
Physician Recruitment and Production Rates and Recruitment-Production Ratios, by County Urban Level—Class of 1960

	Percent Urban Residents (1960)										
	0.00-9.99	10.0-19.9	20.0-29.9	30.0-39.9	40.0-49.9	50.0-59.9	60.0-69.9	70.0-79.9	80.0-89.9	90.0-100.0	Total[a]
Recruitment Rate (RR)[b]	0.27	0.38	0.49	0.59	0.89	0.89	1.07	1.25	1.51	1.63	1.23
Production Rate (PR)[c]	0.91	0.61	1.14	1.18	1.30	0.96	1.44	1.52	1.60	2.27	1.61
Ratio of RR to PR	0.30	0.62	0.43	0.50	0.68	0.93	0.74	0.82	0.94	0.72	0.76

Sources: AAMC Longitudinal Study and U.S. Bureau of Census (1952, 1953; 1967; 1973a; 1973b).

[a]Totals for physicians: 2,418 for county of practice (for recruitment rate) and 2,363 for county or origin (for production rate). Totals for population: 196,730,000 for computing recruitment rate and 146,671,280 for computing production rate (see "County Urban Index" this chapter for explanation).

[b]Number of physicians by county of practice per 100,000 population in 1970.

[c]Number of physicians by county of origin per 100,000 population in 1950.

counties to recruit fewer physicians than they produced, the most urban counties to recruit about the same as they produced, and the middle levels to recruit more than they produced—holds even when population is standardized.

Combined Effects of Income and Percent Urban

The combined effects of income and urbanization on the discrepancies between the number of physicians recruited and produced can be seen by observing the ratio of the number recruited to the number produced for different income-urban county combinations. Since results have shown that the discrepancies in Figures 5-1 and 5-2 are not due to greater population increases in higher income and urban counties, analysis is for absolute numbers. If the ratio of physicians produced to number recruited is 1.00 for a group of counties, the group got exactly as many physicians as it produced; and, of course, if the ratio is above or below 1.00 the number recruited is greater or less than the number produced. Table 5-3 gives the results.[f]

The lowest value is for counties with less than $4,000 annual family income and with less than 40 percent of their population living in urban areas; these counties recruited only 29 percent of the physicians they produced, getting only 40 physicians from the 1960 class but producing 137 of them. The highest values are for counties with $7,000 median family income and above with between 80.0 percent and 89.9 percent of their population living in urban areas; these areas got 3.53 times the number of physicians they produced.

The matrix can also be viewed in terms of the effects of income and percent urban each with variation of the other restricted. For example, the top row includes only counties with at least 90 percent urban residents, thus restricting variation on the urban index but counties that represent several income levels. Thus, comparisons within rows indicate the effect of income with percent urban controlled. Similarly, comparisons within columns indicate the effect of urban for counties of a common income range. Results suggest that the effects of income may be stronger than those of urban. In each of the bottom two rows there are a total of six comparisons between counties of different income levels and 10 comparisons for the top three rows, for a total of 42 comparisons. Although a few of the cells have only a few cases, it is clear that the recruitment-production ratios within each row increase as county income increases. For example, for

---

[f]The total number of physicians in Table 5-3 is 2,249, which is less than the totals on which Table 5-1 and 5-2 are based (2,418 and 2,363/2,361). The explanation is that Tables 5-1 and 5-2 require knowledge of only the income *or* urban level of counties of origin and practice. Table 5-3 requires that both the income and urban level of counties of origin and practice be known.

Table 5-3
Ratio of Number of Physicians Received to Number Produced, by Median Family Income of County and Percent of County Residents Living in Urban Areas—Class of 1960

Percent Urban Residents (1960)	Median Family Income (1959)					
	Less Than $4,000	$4,000-$4,999	$5,000-$5,999	$6,000-$6,999	$7,000 and Over	Totals
90% and above	0.42 (8:19)[a]	2.17 (63:29)	0.73 (248:340)	0.88 (392:447)	1.35 (278:206)	0.95 (989:1041)
80%-89.9%	0.64 (7:11)	0.95 (56:59)	1.26 (87:69)	1.17 (150:128)	3.53 (166:47)	1.48 (466:314)
60%-79.9%	0.42 (8:19)	0.85 (47:55)	0.96 (154:161)	1.58 (153:97)	3.36 (37:11)	1.16 (399:343)
40%-59.9%	0.61 (34:56)	0.73 (46:63)	1.12 (106:95)	1.20 (54:45)	—	0.93 (240:259)
Less than 40%	0.29 (40:137)	0.57 (47:82)	0.80 (36:45)	0.79 (32:28)	—	0.53 (155:292)
Totals	0.40 (97:242)	0.90 (259:288)	0.89 (631:710)	1.05 (781:745)	1.82 (481:264)	1.00 (2249:2249)

Sources: AAMC Longitudinal Study and U.S. Bureau of Census (1967).
[a]Figures in parentheses are N's.

counties with 90.0 percent and more of their residents living in urban areas, the highest income category has the highest ratio in nine out of 10 comparisons. For all rows, counties with the highest income have the highest ratio in 38 out of 42 comparisons; the probability of this occurring by chance is less than 1 time in 100,000. Differences for percent urban with income level restricted are less consistent. For example, for the first, second and fourth columns, for which there are 10 comparisons each, ratios are higher for the higher urban group in only 5 out of 10 comparisons per column. Overall, in 26 of 42 comparisons the higher urban group has a higher ratio than the lower urban group; this would occur by chance about 12 times out of 100. Nevertheless, the lowest and highest ratios are clustered at the extremes on both variables. Counties with high income and high urban values get far more physicians than they produce whereas low-income, rural counties get far fewer than they produce.

A pattern indicated in Table 5-2 is again reflected in Table 5-3. This is that the more urban places get a smaller proportion of the physicians they produce than places with somewhat lower percentages of urban residents. This pattern will be discussed in the next chapter.[g]

The General Process

The process reflected in the relationships of county income and urbanization to physician recruitment-production ratios reflects a general process. A number of observers have commented on the nature of migration patterns from deprived to prosperous areas, although usually expressing the issue in terms of a rural to urban movement. As early as 1924, Edward A. Ross remarked that migration in the United States "has worked on our old rural population like a cream separator," in which the industrious and intelligent persons leave while the lazy and dull stay behind (Ross 1925, pp. 23-24). While the statement may be overdrawn, the general thesis appears to be correct. Evidence based on census data shows that persons who migrate across counties and noncontiguous states, in comparison to nonmigrants, have higher educations, possess more technical occupational skills (e.g., a higher proportion of migrants are classified as "professional and technical"), and earn higher incomes (Bogue 1969, pp. 769-71). These patterns probably hold for persons who migrate from rural economically depressed areas to more affluent areas. Studies by C. Horace Hamilton (cf. 1965) have shown that among persons in younger age groups, who are far more apt than older persons to migrate, migration from rural to urban areas is highly selective of persons

---

[g]Note that this pattern is not detected merely by observing the relationship between urban levels of community of origin and community of practice, as in Table 4-1 of Appendix C. The pattern becomes apparent from a comparison of the marginal distributions for origin and practice (which is what the recruitment-production ratios are) rather than the observation of the relative frequencies of the internal cells.

with better educations. Such a pattern is consistent with the impression gained by natives and authorities on particular rural and economically depressed areas; Harry M. Caudill, a native and authority on Appalachia, writes that historically "waves of out-migration drained off the strong and energetic" from the region and even today the "new vocational schools supply plumbers and typists to many cities in other states" (Caudill 1973, pp. 17, 19). Results in this chapter show that physician talent from rural and poor communities is also drained off and that rural and poor communities help to supply the more urban wealthy communities with physicians as much as they help to supply themselves.

Conclusion

The objective of the past four chapters has been to identify some of the general processes in the maldistribution phenomenon that are the result of nonmedical characteristics of communities. To this end, analysis has shown that the maldistribution of physicians is characterized by two general causal patterns: One is that physicians from all backgrounds tend to locate in higher income urban communities more than in lower income rural communities. The other is that communities which tend to attract more physicians tend also to produce more, and because of the tendency to return to communities similar to the ones in which a person is reared, county differences in production rates reinforce the maldistribution of physicians. The underlying causal processes of these two patterns are related although there are specific differences.

The process contributing to the first pattern is the result of the mutual dependence of the local economy, population base and occupational-service sector along with the linkage of each of these to the extracommunity context. It is probable that this pattern reflects the tendency for physicians to seek environments that provide most in the way of occupational and job opportunities, as well as greater social and cultural opportunities for themselves and their children. The focus, however, should not be exclusively on the motivations of physicians or to imply that these are any different from most other occupational groups. Focus should also be on the characteristics of communities, the reasons why communities differ in these characteristics and the interrelationship between the above three factors. It is within this context that physician migration patterns (and the motives to migrate) occur, and resemble that of other persons with higher educations and technical occupational skills. The educational selectivity (and probably also occupational selectivity) in rural-to-urban migration is not just a rural-to-urban movement; it is a movement from places where occupational opportunities do not exist to places where they do exist (Hansen 1970). Thus "the movement . . . may properly be interpreted as a long-run differential arising from . . . differential rates of economic growth in rural and urban areas" (Bogue 1969, p. 797).

The process contributing to the second pattern derives from community differences in educational and socialization mechanisms associated with differences in income level and urbanization. Although the motivation to return to communities similar to those in which one was socialized is involved, the motivation is, nevertheless, shaped by the nature of the institutions, occupational structure, and culture of the communities in which physicians were reared. Moreover, the influence of this motivation is constrained by the processes involved in the first pattern—the tendency to locate in high-income, urban environments. The result is that low-income, rural communities receive even fewer physicians than they produce. Consequently, they help to supply physicians for wealthy, urban areas more than high-income, urban areas help to supply physicians for them.

A third pattern is also reflected in the results. In the present chapter it was seen that the most urbanized counties as well as the most rural counties get fewer physicians than they produce, with counties between the extremes getting the highest percentage of those they produce. These patterns are largely due to suburbanization, which is the subject of the next chapter.

6 Community Size and Suburbanization

One of the most important social and demographic developments in the United States during the twentieth century has been the emergence of suburbs. This is typically viewed as a movement out of the center of highly urbanized areas to the fringes by middle- and high-income persons. The importance of this movement is reflected in the hundreds of movies, documentaries, journal columns, novels, and social science research studies that have been devoted to it. Considering its apparent importance, it would be most surprising if it were not related to the maldistribution of physicians. This is especially true since the movement occurs in highly urbanized areas. To gain some perspective it will be well to view suburbanization in the context of the framework presented in Chapter 3.

Suburbanization might appear to fall beyond the purview of that framework. This is because the framework focuses on where people work rather than where they live, whereas suburbanization is largely a matter of where people live. Indeed, some suburban communities are called "bedroom communities," which refers to people living in a community but working elsewhere, namely, in the nearby city. Most of the current concern about the suburbs focuses on the residential flight from the cities by the professional and middle class, thereby leaving the inner city to lower income groups. It is probable that the practice settings of physicians have been influenced by the process.

Suburbanization effects members of different occupations in different ways. For some, the suburbs are places to live and work; for others they are places to live only. Workers who are tied to industrial and other organizations are more apt to find employment only where these organizations are located. And for reasons outlined in Chapter 3 these organizations are apt to be located in places where the population is both large and dense. However, the development of transportation and easier access into the city, along with the increased affluence that makes the cost of commuting to the city bearable to a larger proportion of workers, allows people to work in the city and live in communities outside the city. The increased costs of commuting to work in the city is not a barrier to the location patterns of industry. "Calculation in terms of market costs alone do not force the enterprise to take into account the costs of roads and other transport to the factory site, which are paid for by the employee or by the community as a whole out of taxes" (Bell 1962, p. 231). Hence, although members of many occupational groups may live in the suburbs, their work settings remain in the city proper. Given the means of transport and the ability of the worker (and community) to afford that transport, the location patterns of places of work and the workers' movement to the suburbs continue to reflect the reciprocal tie between place of work and residence: Industries locate where they have access to workers and workers live in close proximity (as measured in time and dollars rather than physical space) to places of work. There are physical limits beyond which the commuting distance cannot expand, of course. Consequently, commuting frequently occurs within the boundaries of single counties.

For workers who provide a direct service to the public, the relationship between place of work and residence is different. Their jobs are tied closely to where people live. As Wilbur Thompson's quote in Chapter 2 indicates (see p. 30), location patterns of the service industry are more sensitive to the physical clustering of people than are other industries. Consequently, the location of places of work for physicians (and other professions that provide a direct service to the public) should follow the residential movement of much of the work force to the suburbs. Some of the results in the last chapter suggested this. In this chapter data are presented that provide more definitive evidence.

Previous analysis of physicians in the AAMC Longitudinal Study has been based on characteristics of the counties in which physicians' places of origin and practice are located. Here analysis is based on characteristics of the places themselves. Specifically, differences in recruitment and production of physicians by size of place will be investigated. This will permit an examination of the impact of suburbanization on the practice location of physicians.

The procedure used is similar to that used in examining differences in the recruitment and production rates for counties of different income and urban levels. Of the original 2,514 physicians, the place of origin could be located for 2,308 in the 1963 Rand McNally *Road Atlas for Canada, the United States and Mexico*; the place of practice for 2,359.[a] The population for 1960 as reported by Rand McNally is used to classify physicians as to size of place of origin and practice.

On the basis of 2,308 physicians whose place of origin is known, the number of physicians recruited per 100,000 U.S. population for 1950 is 1.57, and on the basis of 2,359 physicians whose place of practice is known, the number of physicians recruited per 100,000 population for 1970 is 1.20. The ratio between the recruitment rate and production rate is 0.76. The recruitment and production rates and the ratio between the two for the total population provide baselines for assessing differences by size of place. For example, if places of less than 5,000 have a production rate of less than 0.76 they would have produced less than their proportionate share of physicians.

---

[a]Several well-known suburban communities were reported as place of origin or practice but population figures are not available because they are un-incorporated places of urban areas. Consequently, suburban communities are probably underpresented in the analysis.

In Table 6-1, size of place varies from less than 5,000 to 1,000,000 and over. The first row gives the recruitment rate for places of various sizes while the second row gives the production rate. The third row gives the ratio of recruitment to production rates. The way recruitment and production rates are computed for each size category may be seen by way of example.

The number of physicians who were practicing in 1972 in places that had less than 5,000 residents in 1960 was 200. On the basis of figures from the U.S. Census, there were a total of 75,544, 320 persons living in these places in 1970 (U.S. Bureau of the Census, 1973b, p. 18). Dividing the number of physicians (200) by the total population (75,544,320) and multiplying by 100,000 gives the number of physicians per 100,000 total population living in places of 5,000 and less. This is 0.26 (see first row and first column in Table 6-1). In the second row, the number of physicians produced by counties in each of the size categories is expressed as the number of physicians who came from each size category per 100,000 population living in the category in 1950. For example, in 1950, 66,882,102 persons were living in places that had less than 5,000 residents (U.S. Bureau of the Census, 1973b, p. 18). Since these places produced 291 of the physicians in the class of 1960, they produced 0.43 physicians per 100,000 population. For places of less than 5,000 population, the recruitment-production ratio is 0.60.

Results thus permit three comparisons. The first row demonstrates that the recruitment rate is especially low for the smallest communities and tends to increase continuously up to the largest category (cities of 1,000,000 and over), at which point it drops off precipitously. The second row indicates a similar trend for the production rate, except that the drop for the largest places is not as great. The third row reveals that the recruitment-production ratio more or less systematically increases from the smallest communities through communities with 500,000 to 999,999 population. The largest cities, those with 1,000,000 and more residents, have the lowest ratio of any category, which means they got a smaller percentage of the physicians they produced than even the smallest places. Further analysis shows, however, that the difference in the percentage of physicians practicing in these places to the percentage of the total population living in them in 1970 is not extremely large. In 1970, 9.2 percent of the population was living in cities with 1,000,000 and more population (U.S. Bureau of the Census, 1973b, p.18), and this is only slightly more than the 7.9 percent of all physicians from the class of 1960 who were practicing in these places in 1972. Hence, although large cities got a comparatively small proportion of the number of physicians they produced, they still got 85.9 percent (8.3:9.2) of their proportionate share of this cohort of physicians, based on their share of the total population.

Three conclusions are indicated. First, the very large cities have begun to experience some of the same physician manpower problems that poor rural areas have experienced for many years. Indeed, cries are being heard that the supply of manpower in our inner cities is too low to meet the medical needs

Table 6-1
Physician Recruitment and Production Rates and Recruitment-Production Ratios, by Size of Place—Class of 1960

	Size of Place (1960)								
	Less Than 5,000	5,000- 9,999	10,000- 24,999	25,000- 49,999	50,000- 99,999	100,000- 249,999	250,000- 499,999	500,000- 999,999	1,000,000 and Over	Totals[a]
Recruitment Rate (RR)[b]	0.26	1.15	1.71	1.92	1.82	1.89	2.32	2.77	1.03	1.20
Production Rate (PR)[c]	0.43	1.81	1.77	2.03	2.68	2.71	2.40	3.66	2.89	1.57
Ratio of RR to PR	0.60	0.64	0.97	0.94	0.68	0.70	0.97	0.76	0.36	0.76

Sources:　AAMC Longitudinal Data, Rand McNally (1963), and U.S. Bureau of the Census (1973b).

[a]Number of physicians in which population of place of practice is known is 2,362 (for recruitment rate); number in which population of place of origin is known is 2,309 (for production rate). Totals for population: 196,730,000 for computing recruitment rate and 146,671,280 for computing production rate (see this chapter for explanation).

[b]Number of physicians by size of place of practice per 100,000 population in 1970.

[c]Number of physicians by size of place of origin per 100,000 population in 1950.

in these areas. Considering that such cries were seldom heard prior to 1960, it is likely that the situation as reflected in Table 6-1 may have worsened in the past several years.

Second, since large cities receive a much smaller percentage of the physicians they produce than other communities, they appear not even to be attractive to physicians who were reared in large cities. Indeed, results in the third row of Table 6-1 indicate that large cities are even less attractive to their native physicians than the smallest communities are to their native physicians. Still, as noted, the large cities get over 85 percent of their proportionate share of physicians, based on their share of the total population.

Third, a major reason large cities get this many physicians is that they produced such a high proportion; 20.7 percent of all physicians originated from places of 1,000,000 and more. If this percentage decreases in the future, or if it has already decreased since 1960, the proportion of physicians received by large cities to those produced will decrease accordingly. It will be suggested below that this has happened as a result of growth in the suburbs.

Results in Table 6-1 have an important implication for studies concerned with the effect of community size on level of physician manpower. Note the very large difference between cities in the 500,000 to 999,999 range and cities above 1,000,000. Unless a distinction is made between these two categories, studies may come to misleading conclusions concerning the effects of community size on the distribution of physicians. For example, Weiskotten and associates report that communities of 500,000 and over had, in 1959, approximately 18 percent of all 1950 graduates of United States medical schools. They also report that these communities had a much larger proportion of the 1930 graduates (28.9%), and the percentage decreased continuously thereafter for the classes of 1935, 1940, 1945, and 1950. (Weiskotten et al. 1960, pp. 1088-98.) Results in Table 6-1 suggest that the decrease has occurred in the largest cities of this group rather than in those cities in the 500,000 to 999,999 population range.

The results in Table 6-1 bear on suburbanization in a tangential way only. Community variation in the recruitment-production ratio only reveals a movement out of the large cities by physicians who were reared in cities; but they do not show that a large proportion of these physicians established their practices in the suburbs. Since Table 6-1 does not classify communities as suburban or nonsuburban, it is not possible to know the effects of suburbanization directly from the results. The proportion of the population living in suburban areas is substantial. Also, the U.S. Census reports that 7.5 percent of the population lived in unincorporated parts of urbanized areas in 1970 (U.S. Bureau of the Census 1973b, p. 18); and in Table 6-1, these places are included with communities of less than 5,000, as they are in the Weiskotten study,[b] many of which are

---

[b]Compare the figures reported by Herman G. Weiskotten et al. (1960, p. 1088) and by the U.S. Bureau of the Census (1973b, p. 18).

in rural areas. This obviously makes communities in the less than 5,000 size range heterogeneous with respect to their setting—some are in rural areas, and some are in urban areas and hence suburban in character. Consequently, Table 6-1 may underestimate the severity of the manpower problem in small rural communities (this assumes of course that the supply of physicians in suburban communities is higher than it is in communities of comparable size that are located in highly rural areas). The problem is not limited to the very small communities, however; it probably exists for communities up to 50,000 and perhaps to as high as 100,000. Many of these communities are characteristically suburban while others, particularly those in the 5,000 to 24,999 size range, are located in areas that are primarily rural. Still others are located in areas that are neither highly urban nor highly rural. If suburbanization has had an influence on the location patterns of physicians, physician manpower should be higher for small and medium communities in urban areas (the suburban communities) than in the same size communities in more rural areas.

This suggests the following suburbanization hypothesis. The effects of community size on the supply of physician manpower varies depending on the urban level of the surrounding area. Physicians are more apt to be attracted to smaller communities in urban counties but larger communities in rural counties. Community size and urbanization interact.

Suburbanization as Interaction Between Urbanization of County and Community Size

It is possible to test this hypothesis, and in the process correct for the heterogeneous nature of some of the community size categories, by cross classifying physicians by urban level of counties and by size of place within counties. The typical suburb is located near a large city and within a highly urbanized area. Consequently, it is within the more urbanized counties that suburbanization has occurred. Since most suburban communities usually range from unincorporated places of a few hundred to upwards of 50,000 and more, the concentration of physicians in places in this size range would be expected in the most urbanized counties. Unfortunately, the U.S. Census does not report the population of communities by urbanization level of their counties. Consequently, the percentage of physicians who practice in various community size-county urbanization combinations cannot be compared with the corresponding percentage of the total population such as was done for community size in Table 6-1. The ratio of number of physicians received to the number produced for different community size-county urbanization combinations can be computed, however. This will give an index of the overall attractiveness of the places for medical practice. It is assumed that places recruiting more than they produce are most attractive, and hence have relatively high physician-to-population ratios, whereas those recruiting fewer than they produce are least attractive and have relatively low ratios. The recruitment-production ratios for communities of different size ranges located in counties of varying levels of urbanization are presented in Table 6-2.[c]

The ratio in each cell is a function of the numbers in the parentheses in each cell. The first number in the parentheses is the number of physicians recruited by communities in a common size range located in counties of a certain urbanization range. For example, communities of 1,000,000 and more in 1960 located in counties with 95.0 to 100.0 percent of the residents living in urban areas in 1960 recruited 148 physicians from the class of 1960 (cell for top row, last column). The second number is the number of physicians produced; thus, communities with 1,000,000 and more residents in counties with 95.0 to 100.0 percent urban residents produced 372 physicians. The figure above the parentheses is the ratio of the number recruited to the number produced, which in the current case is 0.40. This means that these communities got only 40 percent of the number of physicians they produced.[d]

In making the comparisons in Table 6-2 a problem is created because county urban level and community size are related. For places of origin the product-moment correlation is 0.39; for place of practice the product-moment correlation is 0.27.[e] Consequently, there is a tendency for the largest number of physicians to fall in cells in and around the diagonal. Since small numbers are apt to produce unreliable results, recruitment-production ratios are reported only if there are at least 20 physicians (received and produced combined) in the cell.[f] As a result several cells in Table 6-2 are empty.

In spite of this, the trend is clear. For the more rural counties (those below 60.0% urban residents) the ratio tends to increase as community size increases. On this basis, the larger the community in rural counties, the more attractive it

---

[c]A few communities were located in more than one county that differed in level of urbanization. For example, Chicago is in both Cook and DuPage counties, in which percentage of urban residents are 99.7 percent and 95.3 percent. In these instances the urban level of the county was given the average value. (The same procedure was followed for income values below.)

[d]A distinction is made within the 90.0 to 100.0 percent interval because examination reveals significant differences by community size depending on whether they are in counties with 95.0 percent urban residents and above. This distinction is of little significance for the results based only on county differences.

[e]Inspection of scatter diagrams indicates that the relatively small correlation coefficients are due largely to the fact that the relationships are curvilinear, with a substantial proportion of smaller communities located in urban counties with between 90.0 percent and 100.0 percent urban residents. Gamma coefficients based on categories in Table 6-2 are significantly higher. They are 0.54 for places of origin and 0.78 for places of practice.

[f]This decision is arbitrary. However, data are reported in such a way that the reader can use higher cut-off points if he wishes.

Table 6-2
Production-Recruitment Ratios for Size of Place and Percentage of Urban Residents in the County in Which Place is Located—Class of 1960

Size of Place within County (1960)	Percentage of Urban Residents in County (1960)							
	Less Than 40.0%	40.0-49.9%	50.0-59.9%	60.0-69.9%	70.0-79.9%	80.0-89.9%	90.0-94.5%	95.0-100.0%
1,000,000 and over	a	a	a	a	a	a	0.34 (38:112)[b]	0.40 (148:372)
500,000-999,999	a	a	a	a	a	1.31 (68:52)	0.76 (99:131)	1.21 (174:144)
250,000-499,999	a	a	a	a	a	1.36 (68:50)	1.92 (50:25)	0.89 (100:112)
100,000-249,000	a	a	a	2.67 (16:6)	0.66 (43:65)	0.91 (100:110)	1.25 (36:32)	1.88 (62:33)
50,000-99,999	a	a	1.00 (10:10)	0.70 (30:43)	1.81 (78:43)	1.30 (86:66)	0.65 (11:17)	1.62 (76:47)
25,000-49,999	a	1.84 (35:19)	2.05 (43:21)	1.15 (53:46)	1.20 (48:40)	2.73 (41:15)	2.22 (20:9)	5.29 (90:17)
10,000-24,999	1.09 (35:32)	1.02 (46:45)	1.61 (50:31)	1.13 (36:32)	1.22 (33:27)	4.06 (65:16)	5.06 (28:5)	3.47 (59:17)
5,000-9,999	0.44 (28:63)	1.07 (29:27)	0.47 (8:17)	1.89 (17:9)	1.70 (17:10)	2.63 (21:8)	a	4.50 (18:7)
1,000-4,999	0.50 (64:127)	0.26 (10:38)	a	1.00 (11:11)	2.29 (16:7)	4.67 (28:6)	a	5.67 (17:3)
Less than 1,000	0.19 (10:56)	a	a	a	a	a	a	a

Sources: AAMC Longitudinal Study, U.S. Bureau of the Census (1967) and Rand McNally (1963).

[a] Two few cases to be reliable.   For explanation, see "Suburbanization as Interaction Between Urbanization of County and Community Size," this chapter.
[b] Figures in parenthesis are the number of physicians recruited : number of physicians produced.

is to physicians. Beginning with counties with 60.0 to 69.9 percent urban residents, the relationship begins to shift. No particular pattern is evident by community size for counties in the 60.0 to 69.9 percent urban range. Then beginning with the urban range from 70.0 to 79.9 percent, the ratio more or less continuously decreases from the smallest communities to the largest. The ratios for communities of 1,000,000, all of which are in counties in the 90.0 percent and above urban range, are especially low, and much lower than any other community size range in counties with this proportion of residents living in urban areas. Although the small number of cases in some instances indicates caution in drawing comparisons, the ratio for the largest communities in the 90.0 to 94.9 percent urban range is less than one-fifteenth that of the places with 10,000-24,999 population (0.34 to 5.06), and the ratio of the largest places in counties of 95.0 to 100.0 percent urban residents is one-thirteenth that of the ratio for places with populations between 25,000 and 49,999 (0.40 to 5.29) and one-thirteenth that of places with 1,000 to 4,999 population (0.40 to 5.67). Since the typical suburban communities are less than 50,000 and located in highly urbanized areas, it is significant that the higher ratios are for places with less than 50,000 and located in counties with at least 90.0 percent urban residents. There is no general pattern within these counties for places above 50,000 residents. Most sizes above this level recruited substantially more than they produced—except for the very sharp drop for cities with 1,000,000 residents and above, which recruited only 38 percent of the total they produced (34 percent and 40 percent). Although the empty cells make it impossible to compare the effects of the urban variable on the relationship between community size and the recruitment-production ratio throughout the range of urban values, the differences between small to medium communities and very large cities in the most urbanized counties is clear. The effects of suburbanization on the location patterns of physicians would seem to be indisputable.

Still, the significance of urbanization—or the size-density—of an area in physician location patterns is not to be deemphasized. Comparisons across rows indicate that for most community-size ranges the production-recruitment ratio increases as urbanization of counties increases. The rate of increase varies, however, and decreases as size of place increases. It is still distinct for places in the 100,000-249,999 range (the value of 2.67 for places of this size in the 60.0 to 69.9 percent urban range should be considered in light of the relatively few cases involved). It virtually disappears for communities beyond this size range, however.[g]

---

[g]There is a problem in making within-row comparisions that does not exist for comparisons within columns. Within-column comparisons indicate the effects of community size with urban level of the county controlled. In this instance, a characteristic of the county is viewed as a contextual variable for communities within the county. Between-row comparisons assume that community size is the control variable. Since in very few instances would one community encompass an entire county (or include more than one county), community size does not provide a context for urban level of county.

The interaction between community size and urbanization of county on recruitment-production ratios has an important methodological implication. It indicates that conclusions about the effects of community size on physician manpower are to be drawn with great caution. Unless the relationship between community size and measures of physician manpower is specified with reference to the urban context, conclusions about this relationship are of dubious value. Without such specification, the only meaningful conclusions to be drawn from the current results is that communities of 1,000,000 and more are relatively unattractive places for establishing medical practice and that the attraction of communities with less than 10,000 residents is also comparatively weak (see Table 6-1).[h]

Data have a rather ominous implication for the future of physician manpower in cities of 1,000,000 and more. Although Table 6-2 shows that these places got fewer physicians per 100,000 population than all but those communities of less than 1,000 population, they still got 7.9 percent of all physicians, which is not greatly lower than their share of the total population (9.2 percent). At the same time, these communities got only a small proportion of the physicians they produced. Moreover, separate analysis shows that 52.9 percent of the physicians who were practicing in the largest cities in 1972 actually originated from those communities. (See Table C-2 of Appendix C.) The percentage of physicians who come from communities similar in size to the ones in which they were practicing is substantially less for all other size ranges (see underlined diagonal of Table C-2, Appendix C). Large cities had difficulty attracting physicians of all origins and over half of those they did attract were reared in large cities. Consistent with the analysis of the previous section, this means that the major reason large cities got as many physicians as they did was because they produced so many. It is probable that they produced more because their educational systems were superior to those of most other communities during the forties and fifties when physicians in the 1960 class received their premedical school education. Moreover, the kinds of community characteristics that are conducive to youngsters aspiring to and pursuing higher educations and professional careers, as outlined in Chapter 4, were probably more prevalent in large cities during these periods. With the movement of such a large proportion of the urban middle and professional class to the suburbs, these conditions have changed. (The low-quality education provided by the elementary and secondary schools of large cities has been a source of much concern in recent years.) The implication for the future is clear. If large cities are generally unattractive places to establish medicine, and if the ability of their local institutions to produce physicians (and other professionals) has

---

[h]Lest my remarks be interpreted as only a criticism of the works of others, let me hasten to add that the criticism applies also to an earlier work of mine based on data from the AAMC Longitudinal Study (Rushing 1973).

declined as a result of suburbanization, the physician manpower shortage in large cities is apt to grow worse in the years ahead. It is probable that the proportion of physicians recruited by large cities in classes after 1960 has declined significantly. And many of pre-1960 graduates who had established their practices in the cities have undoubtedly moved to the suburbs. Perhaps some physicians from the 1960 class who were practicing in these cities in 1972 will subsequently leave the cities for the suburbs. The results in Table 6-2 may underestimate the magnitude of the problem.

Again the close connection between community recruitment and production processes is indicated. In Chapter 4 it was argued that the same characteristics of counties which serve to recruit physicians also serve to produce them. Characteristics that help communities to recruit physicians lead to the development of community institutions, occupational structures, and an overall community culture which prepare youngsters for higher education and professional careers and encourage and support them as they pursue these goals. When the institutions, occupational structures, and cultural patterns of communities change, the educational and occupational aspirations and achievements of youths can be expected to change also. Specifically, with the movement of more affluent city dwellers to the suburbs, the institutions, occupational structures (as represented by residents of cities and not those who merely work in the city), and overall culture of cities have changed. Viewed from this perspective, it is in the suburban communities where the greatest productivity gains should be registered among graduating classes after 1960. And since productivity and recruitment processes are related,[i] an uneven distribution of physicians between the suburbs and inner cities would seem to be assured for some time to come.[j]

As noted in Chapter 3, county urbanization and wealth are related. This is because counties that are highly industrialized attract industry, which creates jobs, which in turn increases county income. It has also been noted that suburbanization is typically a process involving middle- and upper-class persons. A relationship between community wealth and suburbanization is therefore indicated.

Suburbanization as Interaction Between County Wealth and Community Size

Table 6-3 presents analysis similar to Table 6-2 but with county income

---

[i]The relationship is far from perfect, of course, as was noted in Chapter 4. Also, large cities in highly urbanized counties obviously represent exceptions to the relationship, as we have just seen.

[j]This assumes that the suburbanization process will not be reversed. At the time of this writing, however, the energy crisis is upon us and there is talk about the possible rebirth of the cities as a result. Suburbs require the means of transport at a price that large numbers of persons can afford. A shortage of energy threatens both of these conditions.

replacing percent of county residents living in urban areas. The fact that income and percent urban are correlated for counties ($r = 0.58$ for all 2,958 counties) indicates that the relationship for income would resemble that for percent urban residents. Analysis shows, however, that income level of county is only weakly correlated with size of places within counties (the r for origins is 0.12 and for practice is -0.02).[k] Consequently, differences within income ranges by community size would be expected to be even greater than the differences reported in Table 6-2.

Results are consistent with the expectation. Still, the patterns in Table 6-3 are similar to those in Table 6-2. Recruitment-production ratios almost continuously increase with community size in counties toward the lower income range (below $5,000); they show no clear pattern for the $5,000-$5,999 range, except that communities with residents of 1,000,000 and more have a very low ratio; and they tend to decrease continuously with community size at the upper income levels ($6,000 and above). In general, county wealth and community size interact in the following way: The positive effects of community size on the recruitment-production ratio is inversely related to the wealth of the broader area in which the community is located. Larger communities are more desirable in areas where the economic conditions are relatively weak, smaller communities are more desirable in areas where economic conditions are relatively strong. The former process leaves small economically depressed communities with a shortage of physicians, the latter contributes to a shortage in inner cities and is an aspect of the suburbanization process. The highest ratios are for places of 1,000-49,999 that are located in counties in which annual family median income is $7,000 and above, which correspond to the suburbs. The smallest ratios are in the lower left and upper right cells, corresponding to economically depressed areas and the inner cities respectively.

Therefore, all the results in Table 6-3 are not reflections of suburbanization. Within-row comparisons between counties of different income levels but with places of uniform size range indicate that recruitment-production ratios increase with income for areas of all size ranges up to those with at least 250,000 inhabitants, after which no particular pattern in the ratio by county income is evident.[1] In addition, community size within counties may be negatively correlated with the income of communities within counties, and the concentration of physicians in smaller communities in the highly urban counties may be partly a reflection of this. The point might be lost by easy reference to the suburbanization process.

-----

[k]As for urbanization, one reason for these low coefficients is that the relationship is curvilinear. A substantial proportion of small communities are located in high income counties. Gamma coefficients based on categories in Table 6-3 are higher, being 0.41 for places of origin and 0.11 for places of practice.

[1]An examination of the effects of county income for communities of a common size poses problems of interpretation. The problem is the same as discussed in footnote g.

Table 6-3
Production-Recruitment Ratios for Size of Place and Income Level of County in Which Place is Located—Class of 1960

Size of Place within County (1960)	Median Annual Family Income of County (1959)					
	Less Than $3,000	$3,000-$3,999	$4,000-$4,999	$5,000-$5,999	$6,000-$6,999	$7,000 and Over
1,000,000 and over	a	a	a	0.39 (102:259)b	0.21 (18:84)	0.47 (60:129)
500,000-999,999	a	a	2.40 (24:10)	1.40 (80:57)	0.86 (189:220)	1.73 (45:26)
250,000-499,999	a	a	a	2.23 (42:19)	1.07 (153:143)	1.38 (25:18)
100,000-249,999	a	a	0.92 (33:36)	1.04 (72:69)	1.01 (105:106)	1.88 (45:24)
50,000-99,999	a	a	1.47 (47:32)	0.94 (73:78)	1.08 (76:70)	2.08 (94:45)
25,000-49,999	a	a	1.55 (42:27)	1.47 (100:68)	1.92 (96:50)	6.92 (83:12)
10,000-24,999	a	0.89 (16:18)	0.82 (49:60)	1.46 (105:72)	2.90 (93:32)	5.19 (83:16)
5,000-9,999	0.59 (10:17)	0.44 (12:27)	0.68 (21:31)	0.87 (34:39)	1.53 (29:19)	4.50 (36:8)
1,000-4,999	0.31 (12:39)	0.35 (16:46)	0.63 (30:48)	0.74 (32:43)	1.71 (36:21)	8.75 (35:4)
Less than 1,000	a	0.08 (2:26)	0.29 (7:24)	1.30 (13:10)	a	a

Sources: AAMC Longitudinal Study, U.S. Bureau of the Census (1967) and Rand McNally (1963).

[a]Too few cases to be reliable. For explanation, see "Suburbanization as Interaction Between Urbanization of County and Community Size," this chapter.

[b]Figures in parentheses are the number of physicians recruited : number of physicians produced.

It is not just a movement of former city dwellers to the suburbs that has attracted physicians; it is a movement of a particular sector of city dwellers—the more or less affluent sector. And where this is not the case, physician shortage is to be expected (cf. Star 1971).

At the same time, it is to be noted that the pattern here is not unique to physicians. The process is general. It is not just that physicians have fled the inner city; a substantial proportion of the middle- and upper-class and professionals of all types have fled. Physicians have merely accompanied and followed their class peers in the process. They are more fortunate than most others, however, since they are more apt than members of other occupations to be able to live as well as to work in the suburbs.

Conclusion

This chapter concludes the analysis of general community characteristics on the maldistribution of physicians. It shows the suburbanization process is a significant aspect of the problem and results indicate that the framework in Chapter 3 provides a useful frame of reference for viewing this process. Of course, the motives and individual characteristics of physicians, as well as that of other persons who decide to locate in the suburbs, are also important. But the suburbanization process is itself a social fact that can be considered independently of those motives. As such, it is causally related to the maldistribution of physicians, which is another social fact.

In the next several chapters the effects of factors specific to medicine rather than general to the community are examined. Their influence on the maldistribution of physicians is examined within the context of the general relationships and patterns that has been identified in the last five chapters.

Part II

Community, Specialization, and Hospitals

7

Specialization, Community Wealth, and Urbanization

In this and the next five chapters the influence of two developments within medicine on the maldistribution of physicians is examined. These are specialization and the corresponding dependence of physicians on hospital facilities. Both have been cited as factors primarily responsible for the maldistribution problem and each has been the subject of several investigations (cf. Fein 1967; Joroff and Navorro 1971; Marden 1966; and Reskin and Campbell 1974). In general, investigations seem to indicate that specialists more than general practitioners are apt to be concentrated in large metropolitan areas and in areas where medical and hospital facilities are more abundant but that both types of physicians are more apt to be concentrated in the areas where incomes are higher and where a high proportion of the population is white (see Anderson and Marshall's review, 1974, p. 197; see also Fein 1967). The present focus differs somewhat from that of other studies. Effort concentrates on showing how the influence of specialization and hospital facilities is related to those factors and processes identified in Part I.

Three general causal patterns in the distribution of physicians have been identified: (1) the interrelationships between the three general dimensions of community structure, with physician manpower being one component of one dimension, and the relationship of these to extracommunity processes; (2) the effect of income and urban differences between communities on differential production rates of physicians, as this is generated by differences in socialization institutions, and the tendency for physicians to practice in community settings similar to the ones in which they were reared; and (3) the role of suburbanization. The effect of specialization on the distribution of physicians is examined within the context of each of the patterns in this and the next two chapters. The current chapter deals with the first pattern and the analysis parallels that in Chapter 2. First, however, the historical trend toward specialty practice is reviewed.

Trend Toward Specialization

Herman G. Weiskotten et al. (1960, p. 1082) give the following number of physicians per 100,000 who report being available for general practice in 1959 by year of graduation:

1950	32%
1945	25%
1940	35%
1935	44%
1930	70%
1925	66%
1920	65%
1915	59%

When the issue is posed in terms of the percentage who limit their practice to a specialty, the increase in specialization is even clearer. In 1923 only 11 percent of all physicians are said to have been in limited practice, in contrast to figures of 41 percent in 1957 (Somers and Somers 1961, p. 27) and 50 percent in 1960 (Somers 1968). For those whose primary specialty is something other than general practice, the percentage was 72 percent in 1963, 76 percent in 1968, and 83 percent in 1971 (Haug et al. 1970, p. 68; Roback 1972; Theodore and Haug 1968, p. 7).

A problem with these statistics is that they include among specialists physicians whose degree of specialization is quite varied. For example, limited specialists such as urologists, orthopedic surgeons, and neurologists are included along with more general specialists such as internists and pediatricians. It is possible, therefore, that the percentage increase in medical specialists really reflects an increase in the percentage of physicians classified as specialists whose specialization is still quite general. However, even when internists and pediatricians are added to the general practitioners, the percentage of all physicians who are generalists consistently declined from 1931 to 1965.[a]

1931	1940	1949	1957	1965
94	89	75	60	50

In the AAMC Longitudinal Study, physicians were asked in 1972 to indicate their primary specialty; a total of 64 specialties were mentioned. These were grouped into three major specialty categories: generalists (general practice and family practice); general specialties (general surgery, internal medicine, pediatrics, and obstetrics-gynecology); and limited specialties (one of 58 specialty categories besides the four general specialties). Percentage in each specialty group is as follows:

---

[a]Reported by Rashi Fein (1967). Calculated from the U.S. Public Health Service (1965, p. 103) and the Surgeon General's Consultant Group on Medical Education (1959, p. 85). In these figures, some general practitioners are part-time specialists.

Limited specialties	55.9%
General specialties	30.6%
General and family practice	13.4%
Unknown	0.1%

Even though the various figures are from different sources and are based on the self report of physicians, there is little question as to the historical trend toward specialization or of the overwhelming concentrating of 1960 graduates in specialty practice.

To show that specialization has increased over time does not, in itself, show that this is responsbile for the current unequal distribution of physicians by community income and urban levels. However, the nature of specialization is such that the distribution of physicians would be expected to differ depending on level of specialization. The more specialized the physician, the fewer the number of persons needing his services. This creates the need to locate in areas where one has access to large numbers of potential clients; only then is there a critical mass to support a specialized occupational role. Therefore, a major factor in the inequitable distribution of physician manpower may stem from community differences in the ability to support certain types of practice. Such support is more likely in large densely populated counties, that is, counties with a high percentage of urban residents.

Also, on balance, the specialist's services are more expensive than the generalist's. (This is true for occupations in general.) The more specialized one is, the more training one is apt to have and, as a consequence, there are relatively few persons with whom one must compete in pricing the service. Thus, the specialist may command high fees. Moreover, the medical specialist is more apt than the generalist to treat patients with conditions that are matters of life or death. From the perspective of a particular patient with a particular problem, the specialist is more apt to render a service that is considered of greater value, and this may be a significant factor in the fee he charges.

According to this interpretation, the strength of the relationships reported in Chapter 2 would be expected to be directly related to specialization; they should be strongest for the most specialized physicians. In contrast to generalists, specialists are more apt to be attracted to areas of high population concentration and where patients have the economic means to pay for medical service. The matter is less problematical for generalists, since they treat a wider range of illnesses and, hence, do not require as large a population base for obtaining patients; and the problem of obtaining patients with the economic ability to pay for their services is not as great. In short, problems in finding community settings with the external economies of scale and sufficient wealth to support a professional (that is, medical) service are inversely related to the degree to which the service is specialized. The hypothesis is investigated drawing on three different sets of data.

All United States Counties

Unfortunately, data that are available for all United States counties, based on the 1966 American Medical Association (AMA) data, distinguish only between general practitioners and all types of specialists combined.[b] As noted, since physician specialists vary in degree of specialization, analysis based on the general practitioner-specialist distinction includes some physicians as specialists whose practices are rather general in scope. For example, in 1966 four general specialists—internists, obstetrician-gynecologists, general surgeons, and pediatricians—constituted 44 percent of all specialists (Theodore, Sutter and Jokiel 1967, p. 48). Therefore, to the extent that there are significant differences between physicians within the specialty category, differences between general practitioners and the more limited specialists are probably suppressed in the statistical analysis by the inclusion of some rather general specialists in the specialty category.

Nevertheless, the differences between the general practitioners and all other physicians is clear from the relationship between community income and each of the physician ratios in Figure 7-1. The regression and correlation coefficients are substantially higher for specialists. On the average, an increase of $1,000 median family income is associated with an increase of 14.80 specialists (0.0148 x 1,000) per 100,000 population. Results for the urban index are similar; the correlation and regression coefficients for specialists are 0.48 and 0.904 for specialists in comparison to only -0.02 and -0.0013 for general practitioners. Thus, on the basis of the regression coefficients, an increase of 10 percent in county residents living in urban areas is, on the average, associated with an increase of 9.04 specialists but a slight decrease among general practitioners.

In addition to the differences in the slope of the regression lines and the correlation coefficients between specialists and general practitioners, differences in the point at which the regression line intersects the vertical axis differs between the two groups of physicians. As Figure 7-1 makes clear, the point of intercept (or the *a* coefficient in the regression equation) is substantially higher for general practitioners than for specialists. (The same is true for results based on the urban index.)[c]

---

[b]In the AMA publication (Theodore, Sutter, and Jokiel 1967), figures on physicians are given by "general practice," "medical specialties," "surgical specialties" and "other specialties" by county. However, because of the limited resources available for collating these data as well as the difficulty in knowing how to consider the specialty categories theoretically, it was decided to collect information only for the total number in patient care and the total number of general practitioners in patient care; the differences between these two, then, is the number of all specialists in patient care.

[c]Analysis was also conducted separately for all nine regional divisions of the country. Wide differences between the two groups of physicians in the correlation and regression coefficients obtained for all nine divisions.

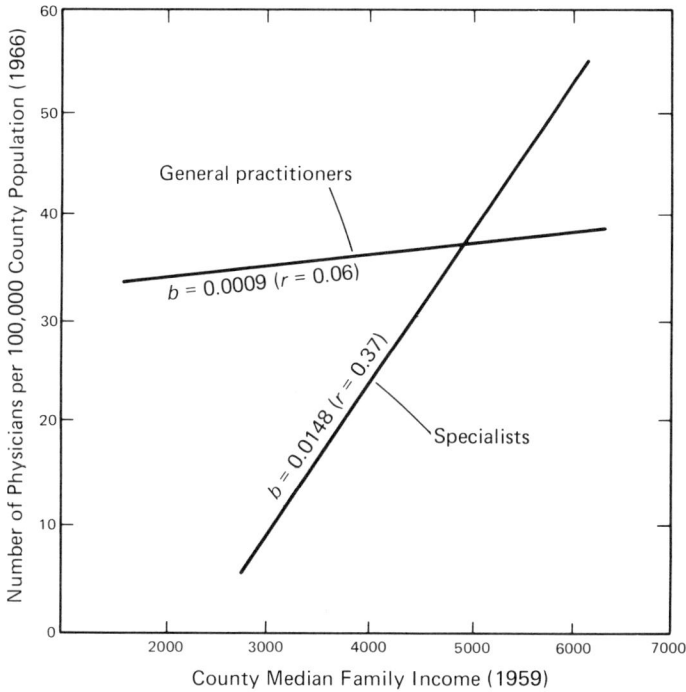

Figure 7-1. Regression of County Physician Ratio on County Median Family Income

These results have the following consequences for communities. Counties with the greatest income advantages are not only apt to have more medical services in general (as indexed by a higher overall physician ratio) and to have at least their proportionate share of general medical services; they are also apt to have a wider range of services as reflected in the results for the distribution of specialists. In addition, to the extent that general practitioners provide the foundation for medical practice as some claim (cf. National Advisory Commission on Health Manpower, Vol. I 1967, p. 25), the foundation appears to be as strong in economically disadvantaged and rural counties as in economically advantaged and more urban counties. In the former there is little else except the foundation, whereas in the latter a large layer of specialty practice is added to the base.[d]

---

[d]The joint effects of county income and urbanization on different types of physicians are examined in Chapter 9.

As noted, the distinction between general practitioners and all specialties masks differences among the latter. If the hypothesis that county income and urban levels are directly related to level of specialization is true, the relationship should differ depending on degree of specialization among specialists. This hypothesis will be investigated for all states and for the class of 1960.

Generalists, General Specialists, and Limited Specialists

For each of the 48 contiguous states, physician ratios are computed for the three major types of physicians (generalists, general specialists, and limited specialists) as of 1971 (Roback 1972), using 1970 as the population base (U.S. Bureau of the Census 1972a). Regression and correlation coefficients are computed between each state physician ratio and the state 1969 median family income and proportion of 1970 residents living in urban areas (U.S. Bureau of the Census 1972b). If the hypothesis is correct, that medical practice is increasingly dependent on urban and affluent environments as level of medical specialization increases, then the slopes of the regression lines should vary depending on level of specialization among specialists. In comparison to limited specialists, general specialists provide either a wider range of services to the community or, as in the case of pediatricians and obstetricians, serve a particularly large proportion of almost any community. Consequently, these specialists are apt to experience less difficulty in obtaining patients who are financially able to sustain their practice. In addition, with the exception of general surgeons, almost none requires referrals from other physicians; contacts with pediatricians, obstetricians, and internists are more apt to be the result of self-selection or of what Eliot Friedson (1960) has called lay referrals. Internists might be somewhat more specialized than the other three because of subspecialties within internal medicine, so that the range of illnesses or problems they treat is more limited than those for pediatricians and general surgeons; also, unlike pediatricians and obstetricians, internists do not provide a service tailored to meet the particular needs of a specific but substantial proportion of almost any community, such as children and women with sex-related medical problems. In any case, steeper regression lines would be expected for all four groups than for general practitioners but not as steep as the regression line for all other specialists (that is, limited specialists).

Results for state income are presented in Figure 7-2. The steepest regression line is for limited specialists, the flattest line for general practitioners, with the lines for the four general specialists between those for the two extreme categories. Differences among specialist categories show that the distribution of internists is more closely patterned on state income than the other three, amongst which there is virtually no difference in slope at all. These results are consistent with the suggestion above that internists are more specialized in their practices than

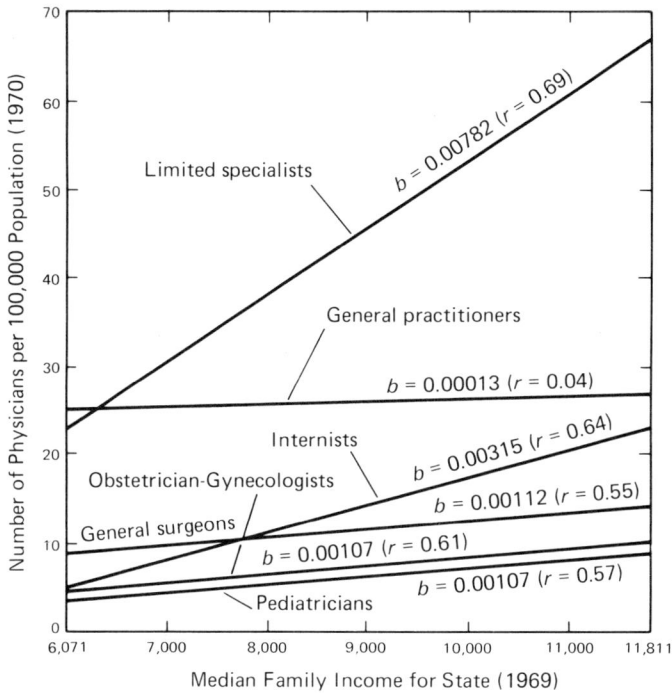

Figure 7-2. Regression of Physician Ratios on Median Family Income (49 Contiguous States)

the other three general specialists. Results for percentage of urban residents are similar (see Table C-3 of Appendix C).

Findings are therefore consistent with the hypothesis that the strength of the relationships between community physician manpower and community income and urbanization are directly related to specialization. Data for states are not exactly for communities, of course, and so they must be accepted with caution. They are, however, consistent with those for all United States counties. They are also consistent with the results for the class of 1960.

Graduates of the class of 1960 are cross classified according to income of county of practice and the three levels of specialization in Table 7-1. To show the association between level of specialization and income of county, a Gamma coefficient is given which is a measure of association between ordinal variables. Although the income measure is interval as well as ordinal, the specialization variable is only ordinal. Limited specialists are more specialized than general specialists, and the latter are more specialized than generalists. There is no basis for assuming, however, that the difference between limited and general

Table 7-1

Relationship Between Median Family Income of Physician's County of Practice and Specialization, in Percentages—Class of 1960

| | Median Family Income (1959) of County of Practice | | | | | |
Specialty	Less Than $4,000	$4,000-$4,999	$5,000-$5,999	$6,000-$6,999	$7,000 and Over	N
Limited specialists[a]	2.1	9.4	28.9	36.1	23.4	1,348
General specialists	3.2	13.0	26.7	33.0	24.1	739
Generalists	15.3	15.9	26.3	28.4	14.1	327

Gamma = 0.16 (x^2 = 141; 8 df; p < .00001)

Sources: AAMC Longitudinal Study and U.S. Bureau of Census (1967).

[a]Percentage does not add to 100 percent because of rounding error.

specialists is equal to the difference between general specialists and generalists; hence specialization is treated as an ordinal variable. The Gamma coefficient is 0.16, which is not very high, though it is statistically significant at beyond the 0.00001 level, based on Chi-square.[e]

Identical analysis is conducted for the urban index. Results in Table 7-2 reveal a relationship that is quite similar to that for income. Counties with higher proportions of urban residents get a higher percentage of both groups of specialists than of generalists whereas counties with the fewest urban residents get a higher proportion of generalists. Therefore, results for the class of 1960 as well as for all United States physicians are consistent with the hypothesis that the concentration of physicians in high income more urban areas is directly related to specialization.

In addition, Tables 7-3 and 7-4 give the ratio of the percentage of each specialty group in counties of different income and urban levels to percentage of total 1970 population living in counties of the corresponding income and urban levels. Ratios are computed in the same way as those for the totals column and row of Table 2-2, except that the ratios are reported separately for each of the specialties. A ratio greater than 1.00 means that counties in the

---

[e]Gamma, of course, is computed from the frequencies rather than percentages. Gamma is known as a "pre" measure, which means that the coefficient indicates the proportion reduction of error obtained when predictions are made for the values of one variable on the basis of knowledge of the values of another. In the present case, the Gamma of 0.16 means that errors of prediction for income of county of practice is improved by 16 percent if predictions are based on specialization of physicians. See Herbert L. Costner (1965).

Table 7-2

Relationship Between Percentage of Residents Living in Urban Areas in Physician's County of Practice and Specialization, in Percentages[a]— Class of 1960

| | Percent Urban Residents (1960) | | | | | |
	Less Than 40.0%	40.0- 59.9%	60.0- 79.9%	80.0- 89.9%	90.0- 100.0%	N
Limited specialists	2.9	9.0	16.9	22.4	48.8	1,346
General specialists	5.7	10.1	18.1	20.7	45.5	736
Generalists	21.2	18.7	20.2	15.0	24.8	326

Gamma = 0.25 (x^2 = 131; 4 df. p < .00001)

Sources: AAMC Longitudinal Study and U.S. Bureau of the Census (1967).
[a]Subject to rounding error.

Table 7-3

Ratio of Percentage of Physicians Practicing in 1972 in Counties of Designated Income Levels to Total 1970 Population of Counties—Class of 1960

| | Median County Income (1959) of Physician County of Practice | | | | | |
	Less Than $4,000 (12.2)[a]	$4,000- $4,999 (14.8)	$5,000- $5,999 (27.5)	$6,000- $6,999 (27.1)	$7,000 and Over (18.5)	N
Limited specialists	0.16 (2.1)[b]	0.64 (9.4)	1.05 (28.9)	1.33 (36.1)	1.22 (22.4)	1,348
General specialists	0.26 (3.2)	0.88 (13.0)	0.97 (26.7)	1.22 (33.0)	1.32 (24.4)	739
Generalists	1.25 (15.3)	1.07 (15.9)	0.96 (26.3)	1.05 (28.4)	0.76 (14.1)	327

Sources: AAMC Longitudinal Study and U.S. Bureau of the Census (1967, 1973a).
[a]Percentage of total 1970 population living in counties in column.
[b]Percentage of physician group practicing in counties in column.

Table 7-4
Ratio of Percentage of Physicians Practicing in 1972 in Counties of Designated Urban Levels to Total 1970 Population of Counties—Class of 1960

	Percentage of Urban Residents Living in Urban Areas (1960)					
	Less Than 40.0% (16.6)[a]	*40.0- 59.9% (14.6)*	*60.0- 79.9% (18.5)*	*80.0- 89.9% (16.9)*	*90.0- 100.0% (33.5)*	*N*
Limited specialists	0.17 (2.9)[b]	0.62 (9.0)	0.91 (16.9)	1.33 (22.4)	1.46 (48.8)	1,346
General specialists	0.34 (5.7)	0.69 (10.1)	0.98 (18.1)	1.22 (20.7)	1.36 (45.5)	736
Generalists	1.28 (21.2)	1.28 (18.7)	1.10 (20.2)	0.89 (15.0)	0.74 (24.8)	326

Sources: AAMC Longitudinal Study and U.S. Bureau of the Census (1967, 1973a).

[a]Figure in parenthesis is percentage of 1970 population living in counties in column.

[b]Figure in parenthesis is percentage of physicians from class of 1960 practicing in 1972 counties in the column.

income (urban) range got more than their proportionate share of physicians, based on their share of the total 1970 population, while a ratio of less than 1.00 indicates that counties got less than their proportionate share. Results for limited and general specialists are consistent with results in Figures 7-1 and 7-2 as well as Tables 7-1 and 7-2, since the ratio increases as county income and urban levels increase. There is a difference for generalists, however, since the ratio decreases from low income and low urban counties to high income and high urban counties. For example, for counties with less than $4,000 annual family income the ratio is 1.25 in comparison to the ratio of 0.76 for counties with $7,000 median family income and above.

Discussion

Medical specialization is clearly an important factor in the maldistribution of physicians. Interpretations in Chapters 1 to 6, which emphasized general community factors as causal in the maldistribution, are more consistent with the patterns for specialists than for generalists, and more consistent with the pattern for limited specialists than for general specialists. Several factors are probably involved. These include community differences in professional associations, cultural and quality of life, and hospital facilities. On balance, however, an interpretation that stresses occupational-economic factors would seem to come closest to accounting for the results. If quality of life factors and social and cultural opportunities were primary, such systematic variation depending on level of specialization would hardly be expected. It is probable that "personal and family preference, quality of schools, cultural activities, . . . and hours of work, etc.," which are viewed as more favorable in urban areas (Fein 1967, p. 75), are just as important to general practitioners as to specialists, and certainly as important to general specialists as to limited specialists. Community differences in hospital facilities probably play a role also, but it could be argued that this is because they increase the income potential for physicians.

Still, economic motives narrowly defined (that is, income maximization) probably do not account for these differences. One survey shows that the average annual net income of one specialty, general surgeons, is $1,700 less in urban areas as in rural areas (Owens, 1970:131). Dr. Harold A. Zintel, an assistant director of the American College of Surgeons, is quoted as saying that many rural communities in need of general surgeons have made houses and offices available but "have been unable to attract a single surgeon" (Owens 1970, p. 132). Differences in the distribution of physicians by specialty are probably more correctly viewed as due to the search for environments that enhance occupational opportunity rather than a search for economic reward per se. If the latter were primary, there would be little reason to expect such sharp differences between communities by level of specialization. Given the belief that the economic demand is so high and the supply of physicians so limited in low income rural communities, it is probable that many specialists could make more money by establishing general practices in these communities. For them to do so, however, would involve a change in occupational career.

It is possible, of course, that different specialties tend to select individuals who have different types of motivations and individual characteristics. Medical students and recent graduates who are most concerned with personal economic enhancement and the culture and quality of the environment may be those most apt to enter specialty practice. In the absence of data in this regard, such a possibility cannot be discounted.

Although occupational-economic motives seem to provide the most general plausible interpretation of differences by specialty, an exclusive focus on individual characteristics presents a limited perspective. The general economic and social characteristics of communities that result in high specialty ratios need themselves to be accounted for rather than be taken as given. The general point was made in Chapter 2. In addition, results in Tables 7-3 and 7-4 show that for the class of 1960 the physician-to-population ratio for generalists is actually higher for low-income, rural areas than it is for urban, high-income areas. In the absence of additional information, this result could hardly be accounted for by motivational factors. The pattern is characteristic only of the class of 1960, and hence may be more typical of recent graduates of medical school rather than of all physicians. The pattern will be examined in more detail in Chapter 9. For the moment it will only be noted that an interpretation that general and family practitioners from the class of 1960 are more strongly attracted to impoverished rural environments than to wealthier urban environments is not correct. These patterns are understandable only in the context of suburbanization.

8

Specialization and the Community Production and Recruitment of Physicians

In Chapter 4 I argued that the county differences in the production of physicians was the result of differences in educational and socialization institutions between counties. I also argued that these were causal factors in the maldistribution of physicians: Physicians tend to practice in counties similar in income and urban characteristics to the one in which they were reared, and the higher income more urban counties are the ones with the highest productivity rates. Hence, high-income, urban counties are best able to attract physicians partly because they produce so many. This may vary, however, depending on physician specialization. The issue is investigated in this chapter.

Specialization, County Origin, and the Production of Physicians

Table 8-1 cross classifies physicians from the class of 1960 by income of county of origin and by type of specialty. Examination indicates that specialists are relatively more likely to originate from high-income counties and generalists relatively more apt to originate from low-income counties. The relationship, while highly statistically significant, is not especially strong, with a Gamma coefficient of only 0.14. But the trend is consistent: The percentage of county physician products who are in limited specialties consistently increases with income level of county of origin (43.6, 53.2, 55.9, 58.5, and 61.6 from poorest to wealthiest county type); the percentage in general specialties shows little variation with county wealth; and the percentage for generalists tends to decrease from poor to wealthy counties (26.5, 16.1, 10.5, 13.2, to 7.8). At the same time, a high proportion of physicians from all county types become specialists (73.6 percent from counties below $4,000 income are specialists). Therefore, results in Table 8-1 reflect two trends: the overall trend toward specialization and the stronger tendency for physicians from wealthier environments to elect to go into specialty rather than general practice. Another study indicates a similar tendency by community size, with students in schools from smaller towns electing careers in general practice (Coker et al. 1960).

Table 8-2 shows the results for urbanization. Results are generally

Table 8-1

Relationship Between Median Family Income of County of Origin and
Specialization, in Percentages[a]—Class of 1960

	Income of County of Origin (1959)				
	Less Than $4,000	$4,000- $4,999	$5,000- $5,999	$6,000- $6,999	$7,000 and Above
Limited specialists	43.6	53.2	55.9	58.5	61.6
General specialists	30.0	30.8	33.5	28.3	30.6
Generalists	26.5	16.1	10.5	13.2	7.8
N	257	299	740	767	294

Gamma = 0.14 (x^2 = 59; 8 df; $p < .00001$)

Source: AAMC Longitudinal Study and U.S. Bureau of Census (1967).
[a]Subject to rounding error.

similar to those for income; the greater the urbanization of the county, the
greater the probability that the physicians produced will be specialists.[a]

The institutional factors responsible for community differences in the
overall production of physicians may account for the differential production
of physicians who follow different specialty careers. Wealthier and more
urban counties generally have better educational institutions that expose students to a more varied curriculum; the tendency to choose more specialized
occupational careers may be encouraged because of this. This in turn may be
reinforced by the life of the community where the individual sees many persons
who are occupational specialists and few persons who have skills that are general to a variety of occupations; communities with highly differentiated occupational structures tend to produce individuals who differ with respect to occupational career lines. Moreover, physician-to-population ratios are usually high
in such communities, and the specialty-physician ratios are especially high.

---

[a]Tables C-4 and C-5 of Appendix C give the ratio of the percentage of each specialty
group from counties of different income and urban levels to percentage of the total 1950
population living in counties of corresponding income and urban levels. Ratios are computed in the same way as those for the totals column and row of Table 4-1, except that
the ratios are reported separately for each of the three specialties. A ratio greater than
1.00 means that counties in the income and urban range produced more than their proportionate share of physicians, based on their share of the total 1950 population, while a
ratio of less than 1.00 indicates that counties got less than their proportionate share.

Table 8-2

Relationship Between Percent Urban Residents of County of Origin and Specialization, in Percentages[a]—Class of 1960

	Percent Urban Residents (1960)				
	Less Than 40.0%	*40.0-59.9%*	*60.0-79.9%*	*80.0-89.9%*	*90.0-100.0%*
Limited specialists	48.1	51.7	54.7	59.1	58.4
General specialists	28.2	30.1	27.8	30.3	32.6
Generalists	23.7	18.1	17.5	10.6	9.0
N	312	259	360	330	1,099

Gamma = 0.24 (x^2 = 60; 8 df; $p < .00001$)

Source: AAMC Longitudinal Study and U.S. Bureau of Census (1969).

[a]Subject to rounding error.

This raises the probability that youngsters growing up in such communities will be exposed to the range of medical careers that are potentially available to them.   In the wealthier more urban counties, educational institutions and occupational structures, mechanisms that are so important in educational and occupational socialization in communities, are more apt to orient youngsters who aspire to medical careers in the direction of specialty careers.

Other factors may also be involved. It is possible that the degree of medical specialization is related to the ability of physicians. The less able students may be more inclined toward general practice careers. Physicians who were reared in poor rural settings, because of their poorer educational backgrounds, may therefore be more inclined to choose general practice as a career.

In addition, selection of a specialty may be influenced by personality factors that are the result of community socialization. Although there are no data on this, general practitioners are popularly viewed as physicians with whom patients may discuss emotional and personal problems that may be unrelated to a specific medical problem, narrowly defined. Some believe that with the decline of general practice, doctor-patient relationships have become too impersonal (see Field 1970). Therefore, some argue there is a need for more general and family practitioners who will inject more warmth, understanding and sympathy in patient-doctor relationships. To the extent that this common conception is true, personality differences may be involved in the relationship between county of origin and specialization. The orientation of

general practitioners to the general medical needs of others may be a reflection
of a more general personal style of interaction with others, which has its roots
in the type of community in which the individual was reared.

It is possible, however, that the relationship between origin and type of
medical career is entirely spurious. The relationship between origin and specialization may simply be a statistical artifact of the fact that each is related to a
third variable. Since Chapter 4 reveals that county of origin is related to county
of practice and Chapter 7 that specialization is also related to county of practice, the relationship between origin and specialization may exist only because
both are associated with county of practice. Findings indicate, however, that
the relationship between county of origin and specialty choice is manifest
before practice in a community begins. During their senior year members of
the 1960 class were asked if they planned to pursue a career in "general practice," "specialty practice," "specialty practice combined with teaching and
research," or "teaching and research." Since the latter does not specify clinical
practice, it will be eliminated from the analysis.[b] Percentages planning each
of the types of careers are as follows: general practice—21 percent; specialty
practice—42 percent; and teaching-research-specialty—37 percent. The percentages vary, however, depending on the income and urban level of county of
origin. Table 8-3 shows the relationship for county income. As can be seen, the
proportion planning a career in general medicine decreases almost continuously
from low-income origins to high-income origins. A similar relationship exists for the
urban index.[c] There is obviously something about growing up in low-income
rural, communities, in comparison to growing up in high-income, urban communities, that psychologically orients individuals aspiring to medical careers
in the direction of general medicine. In this connection, in their study of one
such community, Don Martindale and R. Galen Hanson state that "the individual primarily deals with people one has known all his life and interpersonal
judgments are based largely on detailed knowledge of the individual and his
family" and that the educational and socialization institutions of the community
tend to produce this kind of person (Martindale and Hanson 1969, p. 118-19).
As noted, this is also the kind of person that many people associate with general
practitioners.

In any case, the explanation for differential productivity rates must be in
terms of community structure and institutions. This obviously does not mean
that the process of specialization or the emphasis on specialty practice in medical
education is the result of community institutions outside the field of medicine.
But given the specialization process, the effect of specialization on the type of

---

[b]Only 68 expressed an interest in pursuing a "teaching and research" career.

[c]Gamma for urban, with six groups (less than 50.0%, . . . 90.0-100.0%) and specialization is 0.30 (x^2 = 77; 5 df; $p < 0.00001$).

Table 8-3

Relationship Between Career Plans During Senior Year and Income of County of Origin, in Percentages—Class of 1960

	Income of County of Origin (1959)					
Career Plan	Less Than $3,000	$3,000- $3,999	$4,000- $4,999	$5,000- $5,999	$6,000- $6,999	$7,000 and Over
Specialty[a]	58.6	64.2	71.7	83.6	79.5	86.1
General Practice	41.4	35.8	28.3	16.4	20.5	13.9
N	87	137	254	596	644	238

Gamma = 0.23 (x^2 = 62; 5 $df; p < .00001$)

Sources: AAMC Longitudinal Study and U.S. Bureau of the Census (1967).

[a]Includes plans for combined teaching-research-specialty practice careers.

physician orientation and subsequent medical career will be partly determined by the type of community in which the physician was reared. At the individual level, the relationship between the specialization process in medicine and choice of specialty depends on the individual's community background. I suggest that the mechanism connecting the two is to be found in the institutions of the community in which the physician was reared.

Specialization and the Relationship Between County of Origin and County of Practice

In Chapter 4 it was found that the income and urban level of the physician's county of origin was related to the income and urban level of the physician's county of practice. Since there are wide differences between counties of different income and urban levels in the production of physicians, it was concluded that the production of physicians was a significant factor in the maldistribution of physicians. Although this would indicate that differences in community structure and institutions are significant causal factors in the maldistribution phenomenon independently of community income and urban characteristics that serve to attract physicians, it is nevertheless possible that the relationship between income (urban) level of county of origin and of practice is largely a function of specialization. This apparently would be a conclusion of those who view specialization as the cause of the maldistribution of physicians. It would also be consistent with the bulk of the evidence in the previous chapter. The argument is difficult to refute. Ideally, to show that this is not the case it would be necessary to reduce the proportion of specialists and then see what happens to the distribution of physicians over a period of years.

The problem can be approached from another angle, however. The relationship between income (urbanization) of county of origin and income (urbanization) of county of practice can be examined for each of the three levels of specialization. This permits the study of the relationship in which variation in degree of specialization is limited. Consequently, if the effects of county of origin on location decision are due solely to specialization, the relationships between income and urbanization of county of origin and of county of practice should disappear or be reduced significantly in magnitude for each of the three groups. In Chapter 4 the product-moment correlation and regression coefficients for these relationships for all physicians were 0.39 and 0.352 for county income and 0.29 and 0.227 for urbanization. Corresponding coefficients are presented for each of the three specialty groups in Table 8-4. The regression lines are drawn for county income in Figure 8-1.

For none of the three groups do the coefficients reduce to zero; all r's are significantly greater than 0.00 for both community income and urbanization. This means that the effects of place of origin on selection of place of practice is not due solely to specialization. For all three groups of specialists there is a tendency for physicians to practice in settings similar to the ones in which they

Table 8-4
Relationships Between Characteristics of Place of Origin (O) and Characteristics of Place of Practice (P), by Specialty—Class of 1960

Relationship	Specialty[a]	r[b]	b	a	N
Income$_O$, Income$_P$	LS	0.30	0.264	4,704	1,269
Income$_O$, Income$_P$	GS	0.37	0.341	4,193	701
Income$_O$, Income$_P$	G	0.55	0.528	2,742	311
% Urban$_O$, % Urban$_P$	LS	0.21	0.145	73.0	1,271
% Urban$_O$, % Urban$_P$	GS	0.30	0.235	62.7	698
% Urban$_O$, % Urban$_P$	G	0.30	0.280	46.0	310

Sources: AAMC Longitudinal Study and U.S. Bureau of the Census (1967).
[a]LS = Limited Specialty; GS = General Specialty; G = Generalists.
[b]All correlations are significant at beyond the .00005 level or beyond.

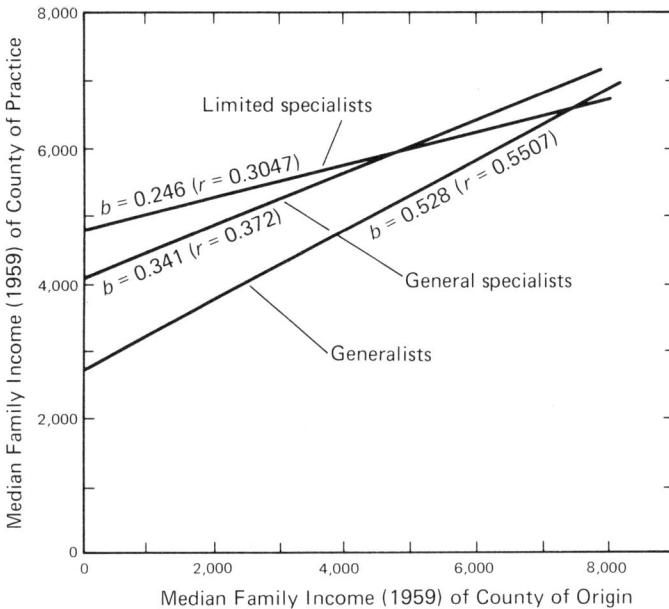

Figure 8-1. Regression of Income for Physician's County of Practice on Income for Physician's County of Origin, by Specialty—Class of 1960

were socialized. Obviously control for specialization does not result in the disappearance of the statistical association between community of origin and community of practice; the effects of community differences in the production of physicians is partially independent of specialization. Consequently, differences in the county production of physicians are significant in the distribution of all three types of physicians, and the types of institutions that contribute to different productivity rates are probably important causes of the maldistribution phenomenon.

At the same time, the results in Table 8-4 and Figure 8-1 also reveal the significance of specialization. It was noted in Chapter 4 that the tendency for physicians from low-income, rural counties to locate in higher income, more urban counties is stronger than the tendency for physicians from high-income, urban counties to locate in lower income, less urban counties. It was also noted that the existence of both tendencies is what kept the coefficients from approching 1.00, and that a coefficient of 1.00—a perfect relationship between origin and practice, in which counties of different income levels got exactly as many physicians as they produced—would make for a more even distribution of physicians than is now the case. Since the coefficients for general and family practitioners more nearly approach this level, generalists are more apt to practice in settings in which they were reared and are thus more evenly distributed across counties of different income and urban characteristics. The same is true for general specialists in comparison to limited specialists. Thus the causes of differential county productivity rates (socialization and educational institutions) and specialization interact in their effect on the maldistribution of physicians.[d]

This would suggest that a focus on specialization as the primary cause of the maldistribution of physicians, which is the case in some circles, is too narrow. The reasons may be seen most clearly in Figure 8-1. Note that it is among physicians from the poorest counties that the differences between the regression lines are greatest. This means that the tendency for general practitioners from poor counties to establish their practices in high-income counties is weaker than the tendency among specialists, and the tendency among general specialists is weaker than it is among limited specialists. The distance between the regression lines decreases as income of origin increases and virtually disappears among physicians from the wealthiest origins. For physicians from the wealthiest counties, those who locate in lower income counties reduce the magnitude of the regression coefficient. As Figure 8-1 shows, there is very little difference between specialties in this respect; the regression lines for the three groups converge. Therefore, general practitioners who come from high-income areas are about as likely to locate in high-income areas as are other physicians. On the basis of these results, then, a reduction in the proportion of physicians entering specialized practice would have little if any effect on the maldistribution problem unless corresponding changes were made in the educational and socialization institutions which differentiate between wealthy urban counties and poor rural counties. (The issue will be explored in detail in Chapter 12.) Again the significance of the community production process as a causal factor in the distribution of physicians is indicated.

---

[d]In Table 8-4, all differences between the correlations for $Income_O$ and $Income_P$ are statistically significant at beyond the .001 level, except the difference between the correlations for GS and G, which is significant at the .10 level. For correlations between % $Urban_O$ and % $Urban_P$, only the differences between LS and GS is statistically significant ($p < .05$), although the difference for LS and G is statistically significant at the .10 level.

9 Specialization and Suburbanization

The analysis of the suburbs in Chapter 6 indicates that the primary impact of the suburbs has been to draw physicians away from the cities. The question arises as to whether the process is more typical of some types of physicians than of others. It has been seen that the attraction of high income and urban counties varies directly with level of physician specialization and that the tendency to practice in counties similar to the counties of origin is strongest for generalists and weakest for limited specialists. There is reason to believe that suburbanization also has a differential impact, depending on physician specialization. General and family practitioners would be expected to be effected more than specialists. This is because the latter are tied more to places where specialized hospital facilities are located, and these are more apt to be in the large cities than in towns and medium cities surrounding the cities. This may have restrained many specialists from moving their practices to the suburbs, or of establishing their initial practices in the suburbs. This restraint is probably not as strong for general and family practitioners. In addition, small suburban communities may not provide the range of external economies that many specialists require, whereas this is not as crucial for general physicians. For these reasons, then, the effect of the suburbs would be expected to be inversely related to level of specialization.

Specialists and General Practitioners

In Chapter 2 the median physician ratio was given for all United States counties cross classified by level of county income and urbanization (Table 2-1). The identical cross classification is presented for general practitioners and specialists separately in Tables 9-1 and 9-2. Results for general practitioners in Table 9-1 are discussed first.

Inspection of Table 9-1 reveals two patterns: One is that most of the differences between cells are not very great, with most values falling between 30 to 40 physicians per 100,000 population. This reflects the pattern for general practitioners to be rather evenly distributed across counties of different income and urban levels. The second pattern is for the effects of urbanization to vary depending on income level. If the cells with very few cases are ignored, the ratio increases as urbanization increases for counties with less than $3,000 median family income (first two columns); there is no trend for counties in the

119

Table 9-1
Median General Practioner Ratio (1966) for 2,958 Counties by Median Family County Income and Percent Residents Living in Urban Areas

Percent Urban Residents (1960)	Median Family Income (1959)					
	Less Than $2,000	$2,000-$2,999	$3,000-$3,999	$4,000-$4,999	$5,000-$5,999	$6,000 and Over
70 and over		27.2 (5)[a]	34.2 (6)	24.6 (58)	27.8 (109)	28.4 (149)
50.0-69.9		39.4 (12)	37.0 (91)	36.1 (146)	34.9 (184)	31.5 (58)
30.0-49.9	43.5 (3)	35.6 (118)	37.6 (175)	38.4 (247)	39.2 (168)	36.4 (25)
10.0-29.9	30.0 (28)	33.0 (124)	36.1 (143)	39.2 (129)	39.3 (57)	26.1 (7)
Less than 10.0	25.8 (81)	26.4 (268)	34.2 (281)	38.5 (206)	39.7 (67)	40.5 (13)

Source: C.N. Theodore, G.E. Sutter, and E.A. Jokiel (1967) and U.S. Bureau of the Census (1967).
[a]Figure in parenthesis is number of counties.

$3,000-$3,999 range; for counties beyond this level, the ratio tends to decrease as urbanization increases and, with the one cell with only seven cases eliminated, the tendency becomes increasely clear as income level increases. (There is also some indication that the effects of county income very depending on level of urbanization, with the ratio increasing with income at low urban levels but decreasing or not changing at all at higher urban levels, but this pattern is not nearly as clear.)

Results are thus consistent with the view that the distribution of general practitioners has been influenced by the suburbs. Where income levels of counties are high, general practitioners are more apt to locate in the less urbanized counties. This assumes, of course, that high-income counties with smaller proportions of urban residents contain more communities that are suburban than high-income counties with larger proportions of urban residents.

Quite a different pattern is indicated for specialists (Table 9-2). The median specialist ratio increases as urbanization increases for counties in all income levels (this is especially clear if cells with small numbers of counties are ignored). Unlike general practitioners, specialists are more apt to be located in the most urbanized counties where income level is high, as well as for counties of other income levels when cells with only a few counties are eliminated. The difference is consistent with the hypothesis that the suburbs have had a greater effect on general practitioners than on specialists.

The pattern for the general practitioner ratio to decrease with level of urbanization among higher income counties is similar to the finding for physicians in the Class of 1960, as reported in Table 2-2 of Chapter 2. Since the latter finding is much clearer than that for all general practitioners in Table 9-1, results suggest that the pattern in Table 9-1 may be largely the result of differences in the distribution of general practitioners in recent years and, therefore, to be the result of suburbanization. Separate analysis for the three specialty groups of the class of 1960 is consistent with this hypothesis.

It was observed in Chapter 2 that the product-moment correlation between income and urban level of counties of practice was 0.45 for all physicians in the class of 1960. Since this correlation corresponds to the cross-tabular analysis of Table 2-2, a correlation higher than this would indicate an accentuation of the pattern observed in that table while a lower correlation would indicate an attenuation of the pattern. Correlations for the three groups are as follows: generalists ($r = 0.56, N = 325$); general specialists ($r = 0.45, N = 733$); and limited specialists ($r = 0.33, N = 1,336$).[a] Construction of tables for each of the three specialty groups similar to that of Table 2-2 poses problems because of the small number of cases entering some of the cells, especially for general and family practitioners, who number only 325. Nevertheless, concentration of

---

[a]All correlations are significantly different from 0.0 at the 0.00001 and or beyond. Differences between all correlations are statistically significant at the .03 level or beyond.

Table 9-2
Median Specialist Ratio (1966) for 2,958 U.S. Counties by Median Family Income and Percent Residents Living in Urban Areas

Percent Urban Residents (1960)	Median Family Income (1959)					
	Less Than $2,000	$2,000–$2,999	$3,000–$3,999	$4,000–$4,999	$5,000–$5,999	$6,000 and Over
70.0 and above		5.57 (5)[a]	7.07 (6)	57.41 (58)	77.80 (109)	84.63 (149)
50.0–69.9		3.63 (12)	22.86 (91)	27.02 (146)	41.41 (184)	35.85 (58)
30.0–49.9	0.01 (3)	10.93 (118)	11.84 (175)	12.12 (247)	22.08 (168)	28.90 (25)
10.0–29.9	7.52 (28)	5.43 (124)	8.03 (143)	8.64 (129)	13.50 (57)	12.11 (7)
Less than 10.0	3.84 (81)	3.03 (268)	1.27 (281)	3.56 (206)	6.30 (67)	6.61 (13)

Source: C.N. Theodore, G.E. Sutter, E.A. Jokiel (1967) and U.S. Bureau of the Census (1967).

[a]Figure in parenthesis is number of counties.

physicians in the less urban counties when income is high and the more urban counties when income is low is inversely related to level of specialization, being strongest for general and family practitioners and weakest for limited specialists. Categories for these tables have been combined (less than $6,000 and $6,000 and over; less than 70.0% urban residents, 70.0-89.9%, and 90.0% and over) and are presented in Tables C-6, C-7, and C-8 of Appendix C.

Specialization, Community Size, and Suburbanization

In Chapter 6 it was seen that the physician manpower varied widely depending on the size of communities within counties. It was also seen that the attractiveness of community size varied depending on the urban and income level of the wider county. Smaller communities were more attractive than larger communities in the more urban (and wealthier) counties, larger communities more attractive in the more rural (and poorer) counties. The first pattern is what would be expected as a result of suburbanization. Analysis similar to that for all physicians is now presented for each of the three specialty groups for the class of 1960.

Table 9-3 gives the median population of physicians' places of practice and places of origin by specialty category and level of urbanization of counties. First, observe the totals column, which combines all three physician groups. (The totals column is another way to summarize findings for production-recruitment ratios in Table 6-2.) As can be seen, the median population for places of practice continuously increases from 4,857 for the least urbanized counties (less than 40.0 percent residents living in urban areas) to 475,542 for counties in which 90.0-94.9 percent of the residents live in urban areas and then increases very slightly (to 482,872) for the most urbanized category. Median size for place of origin also increases continuously from low to high urban counties but the difference in size between the two most urban groups is substantial (604,331 to 939,027). For the class of 1960, then, the larger places (inner cities) in the highly urbanized areas were relatively more important in the production of physicians than in their recruitment.

The greater attraction of smaller places to physicians is not limited to the more urbanized counties, however. This can be seen by comparing the sizes of places of practice with places of origin for all county urban levels. For places in the least urbanized counties (less than 40.0 to 59.9 percent), places of practice are larger than places of origin, whereas just the reverse is the case for places located in the three county groups with the highest proportion of urban residents (at least 80.0 percent). Moreover, for the three most urban groups, the difference between size for place of origin and of practice increases as urbanization of county increases.

Table 9-3
Median Size of Places of Practice and Places of Origin in 1960 by Percentage of Urban Residents in 1960 for County in Which Places are Located, by Specialty—Class of 1960

Percentage of Urban Residents in County		Generalists	General Specialists	Limited Specialists	Totals
95.0-100.0%	Practice	219,948	313,410	493,886	482,872
	Origin	493,923	1,670,097	1,670,136	939,027
90.0-94.9%	Practice	356,450	502,550	356,368	475,542
	Origin	601,958	604,310	604,335	604,331
80.0-89.9%	Practice	44,529	76,671	97,810	91,181
	Origin	91,073	119,484	174,461	144,422
70.0-79.9%	Practice	16,316	46,517	67,339	56,607
	Origin	42,115	48,040	67,342	56,753
60.0-69.9%	Practice	16,974	33,410	37,276	32,851
	Origin	30,419	33,446	33,589	33,443
50.0-59.9%	Practice	13,409	24,590	23,488	22,524
	Origin	13,472	5,833	16,868	15,823
40.0-49.9%	Practice	9,453	13,122	22,860	17,583
	Origin	6,754	8,392	12,741	9,791
Less than 40.0%	Practice	3,659	9,189	8,796	4,857
	Origin	2,584	2,707	3,587	3,219
Totals	Practice	16,075	59,365	97,808	66,676
	Origin	33,161	143,663	186,587	134,393

Sources: AAMC Longitudinal Study, Rand McNally (1963), and U.S. Bureau of the Census (1967).

The patterns reflected in the totals column vary, however, depending on level of specialization. They are more characteristic of generalists and general specialists than of limited specialists. Specifically, whereas the median size for places of practice in the most urbanized counties (95.0-100.0%) is smaller than that for places in the next most urbanized counties (90.0-94.9%) for generalists and general specialists, it is larger for limited specialists (493,886 versus 356,368). For the latter group, median size of place of practice increases continuously as urbanization of county increases. This supports the hypothesis that the more specialized physicians are not drawn from the cities to the suburbs as much as other physicians, although the similarity between generalists and general specialists is somewhat at variance with the hypothesis.

Therefore, the differential impact of suburbanization depending on specialization has a result quite different than does the differential impact or urban and income differences between counties. Because of the latter, rural economically depressed counties have a greater shortage of specialists than of generalists, and a greater shortage of limited specialists than of general specialists. Suburbanization creates the reverse situation for the inner cities, since the shortage is greater for generalists than for specialists, particularly limited specialists. Hence, the things that make urban areas relatively more attractive to specialists than to generalists—their external economies of scale and availability of hospital facilities—also help inner cities to compete better for limited specialists than for the less specialized physicians. The same factors are probably reflected in the differences between the three physicians groups in size of place of practice within levels of urbanization. Within all eight levels in Table 9-3, median size of place of practice is smallest for generalists and in five instances it is largest for limited specialists. Hence, the effect of community size, and presumably the external economies and hospital facilities that are probably associated with it, on physician manpower is directly related to physician specialization.

Although Table 9-3 reveals that the effects of suburbanization are greater for generalists and general specialists, limited specialists have also been effected. This is indicated by a comparison of the median population for place of practice with median population for place of origin within each of the urban levels. For limited specialists as well as the other two groups, the median population for place of practice is smaller than the median population for place of origin in every comparison for counties in the three levels of urbanization with at least 80.0 percent urban residents. Moreover, the size for place of practice relative to that for place of origin tends to decrease for all three groups as level of urbanization increases. Although the effect of suburbanization varies among the three specialty groups, suburban communities provide attractive practice settings for all three.

Results based on analysis identical to that for Table 9-3 is presented in Table 9-4 with county income replacing county urbanization level. It will be recalled that it is the towns and small cities in the wealthiest counties that are

Table 9-4

Median Size of Places of Practice and Origin in 1960 by Median Annual Family Income in 1959 for County in Which Places are Located, by Specialty—Class of 1960

Median Annual Family Income of County		Generalists	General Specialists	Limited Specialists	Totals
$7,000 and above	Practice	10,333	59,364	53,795	52,286
	Origin	47,585	482,873	749,992	750,018
$6,000-$6,999	Practice	42,167	126,708	208,982	166,689
	Origin	220,017	318,612	482,870	405,220
$5,000-$5,999	Practice	21,868	75,408	107,716	75,408
	Origin	63,392	697,196	201,033	201,030
$4,000-$4,999	Practice	7,379	36,642	70,609	35,238
	Origin	8,146	16,635	25,246	18,014
$3,000-$3,999	Practice	4,474	23,632	26,256	15,678
	Origin	6,207	8,356	3,011	4,412
Less than $3,000	Practice	4,106	9,903	7,263	5,434
	Origin	6,207	8,356	3,011	4,412
Totals	Practice	16,075	59,365	97,808	66,676
	Origin	33,161	143,663	186,587	134,393

Sources: AAMC Longitudinal Study, Rand McNally (1963), and U.S. Bureau of the Census (1967).

typically suburban communities. Consequently, if the general suburbanization hypothesis is correct—that physicians in general have been drawn from the larger cities to the suburbs, and if the hypothesis that this effect is restrained more for specialists than for generalists is true, the following results should obtain. The relationship between county income and size of place of practice is curvilinear—with the places in the wealthiest counties being smaller than the places in counties lower in income, but that the curvilinear pattern would be less evident among specialists.

Results in Table 9-4 are consistent only with a general suburbanization hypothesis; there is no evidence of a differential impact depending on level of specialization. As can be seen, the relationship between income of county and size of place of practice is curvilinear for all three groups of physicians; for all three, the size for places of practice is smaller for the wealthiest counties (at least $7,000 annual family income) than for places of practice in the next most wealthy counties (those in the $6,000-$6,999 range). At the same time comparisons between size for places of practice with size for places of origin suggest that the attractiveness of smaller places is greater for generalists and general specialists than for limited specialists. The differences between size of places of practice and origin for counties in the $5,000-$5,999 and $6,000-$6,999 ranges are substantially greater for generalists and general specialists.

In summary, cross classification of size of places with county urbanization and income indicates that suburbanization has had a substantial impact on all three groups of physicians who graduated from medical school in 1960. Evidence that the effect is inversely related to level of specialization is clearer for analysis based on urbanization of county, although some evidence exists for income of county also. Since the overall results suggest that the effects of suburbanization are greater for the class of 1960 than for all physicians, data are thus consistent with the fact that the tremendous impact of suburbanization on American cities began after World War II. Certainly they are consistent with the view that the effects of suburbanization on physician manpower distribution have had a shorter history than those associated with urban and income differences between counties, which have been noted since the early part of the twentieth century. They are also consistent with current claims and cries of alarm that large cities, or at least their inner portions, are now experiencing a physician shortage just as rural economically depressed areas have experienced for several decades. Data suggest a difference in the nature of the shortage, however. In rural and low income areas the greatest shortage is one of too few specialists; in the cities shortages are greatest for generalists and generalist-specialists. However, since general specialists include internists, pediatricians, and obstetrician-gynecologists, as well as general surgeons, both rural, low-income areas and the congested urban centers have shortages of primary-care physicians.

Finally, it was also noted that with urban level of county held constant, size of place of practice is directly related to specialization. The same is true when income of county is controlled; in all comparisons within the six county income levels in Table 9-4, the place of practice is smallest for generalists and in four of six comparisons it is largest for limited specialists. It has been suggested that one factor contributing to these differences is the existence of more hospital facilities in larger communities. The role of hospital facilities in the maldistribution of physicians is examined in the next two chapters.

10

Specialization and the Role of Hospital Facilities: Distributional Aspects

Some believe that differences between communities in physician manpower are due in large part to community differences in hospital facilities and that the equalization of hospital facilities would contribute to the solution of community inequities in the supply of physicians. In this chapter the relationship between physician hospital facilities and physician manpower for all counties in the United States will be investigated. The number of general hospital beds per 100,000 population will be used as a measure of hospital facilities, using data reported by Theodore, Sutter, and Jokiel (1967). Then the interaction between general county characteristics and hospital facilities on the distribution of physicians will be examined.

Specialists, General Practitioners, and Hospital Facilities

The dependence of physicians on hospitals is well known. Although historically physicians treated most of their patients in their offices or in the patients' homes, this was before the days of extreme specialization and the development of many forms of diagnostic and therapeutic technology and support personnel, the expense of which hospitals have generally had to bear. Because of the types of illnesses they treat, specialists are, of course, more dependent on hospital facilities than are general practitioners.

For all 2,971 counties, however, there is very little difference in the degree of association between the hospital-bed ratio and each of the physician ratios; for specialists $r = 0.41$, for general practitioners $r = 0.31$.[a] (Corresponding correlation ratios, η, are 0.44 and 0.35.) Still, analysis based on regression analysis indicates that the statistical effect of hospital facilities on the specialist ratio is approximately four times as great as on general practitioners; b coefficients are 0.0839 and 0.0221. Thus, for each increase of 100 general hospital beds per 100,000 population there is on the average an increase of 8.39 specialists and

---

[a]Ratios for hospital beds are for short-term general hospitals, thus "excluding those classified as federal; long-term; psychiatric, tuberculosis, chronic disease and/or convalescent, and children's hospitals for these categories; and hospital departments of an institution" (Theodore, Sutter, and Jokiel 1967, p. 20).

2.21 general practitioners per 100,000 population.[b] Differences are graphically shown by the regression lines in Figure 10-1. These results are consistent, therefore, with the general observation that specialists are more dependent than general practitioners on hospital facilities. They are also consistent with the belief that one way to attract physicians (especially specialists) to a community is to establish hospital facilities in the community.

A limitation of these results is that they combine units of analysis (counties) that are heterogeneous with respect to a number of factors, especially with respect to level of economic well being and urbanization. It is possible, therefore, that the results in Figure 10-1 conceal wide variation in the relationship between

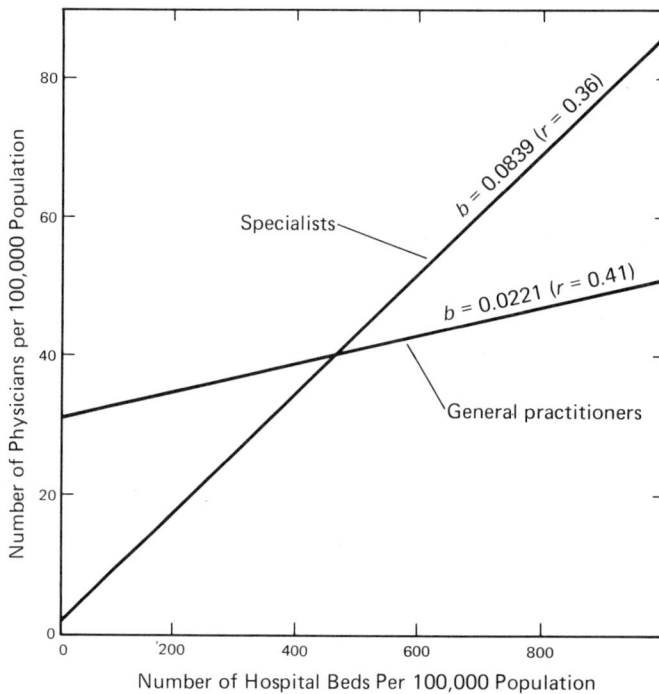

Figure 10-1. Regression of General Practitioner and Specialist Ratios on Hospital-bed Ratios

[b]We note again the possible methodological difficulties when correlations are between ratios that have a common term, such as in the present case where the denominator for physician ratios and hospital bed ratio is county population. (See Appendix A.) We might note here, however, that the presence of a common term in the two ratios does not account for the *difference* in the *b* coefficients between general practitioners and specialists.

hospital-bed and physician ratios for counties of different income and urban levels. There is reason to believe that this is the case. A community's ability to attract physicians with hospital facilities depends to a substantial degree on other community characteristics. Although hospital facilities are probably necessary conditions for attracting physicians (especially specialists) to communties, they are not sufficient conditions. Their ability to attract physicians varies depending on the income and urban level of the community in which the facilities are located. That is, type of community and hospital facilities may interact. However, since general practitioners are less dependent on hospital facilities than specialists, as well as the fact that the distribution of general practitioners is not associated with either county income or urban level, only in the case of specialists would such interactive effects be expected.

Hospital Facilities and Structural Constraints: A Theoretical Statement

The general framework for communities in Chapter 3 emphasizes the interdependence between characteristics of community. It is in terms of this general perspective that the relationship between hospital facilities and physicians (specialists) is viewed. Of course, both physicians and hospitals are aspects of the local service structure and of a subsector (the medical component) of this structure, and for this reason a positive relationship between them would be expected. But within this subsector a distinction between physicians and hospital facilities is made. Hospital facilities are viewed as a form of community capital expenditure and physician manpower as a form of human resource. Hospital facilities are thus viewed from the same perspective that one views highway construction in economically depressed regions or school construction in disadvantaged communities. Sometimes these capital outlays influence human resource development (e.g., better educational facilities may attract more and better qualified teachers), and sometimes they do not. According to Niles Hansen's (1970) analysis, however, such programs (e.g., highway construction) have not been very successful; they generally fail to raise the level of human resources in economically depressed rural regions and communities. The effect of hospital facilities (as indexed by the number of general hospital beds per 100,000 population) may be similar. The extent to which communities are able to attract human resources (physicians) with hospital facilities will depend on more general social and economic characteristics of the community. Therefore community income and urban levels are contextual properties that influence the relationship between hospital facilities and physicians. Put differently, the general economic and urban context of community is viewed as a structural constraint that influences the effect hospital facilities have in attracting physicians to the community.

Alternative Formulation of the Problem

Other studies have consistently shown that the wealth, the percent urban residents, and the hospital-bed ratio of areas are associated with the distribution of physicians. In some studies investigators view the effects of these variables as additive. Although authors are usually careful to indicate that several factors besides hospital beds are involved, such as population size, urbanization, and economic factors, they may tend nevertheless to assume that because hospital beds explain a portion of the variance in the supply of physician manpower that is not explained by other factors, hospital beds have an effect that is independent of other factors (Joroff and Navorro 1971; Marden 1966). The point is explicit in the early work of Joseph W. Mountin, Elliott H. Pennell, and Virginia Nicolay, who state:

> *Regardless* of income class of the county, the presence of a large number of hospital beds reflects more attractive locations for physicians ... Such facilities *alone* afford attraction for establishing medical practice apart from other factors such as wealth, population expansion, and urban character of counties [1942, p. 1952; emphasis supplied] .

The hypothesis here is different. The extent to which hospital facilities and physician manpower are associated is believed to vary depending on the community context.[c]

Hospital Beds, Physicians, and Structural Constraints

In order to study the relationship between hospital facilities and physician ratios under different contextual conditions, communities must be distinguished in terms of context. Five different community (county) types used in the United States Census prior to 1970 are Greater Metropolitan (GM), Lesser Metropolitan (LM), Adjacent to Metropolitan (AM), Rural (R) and Isolated Rural (IR). Although these five are selected largely because they are readily available, distinctions between them correspond to significant differences in levels of county income and urbanization. The five county types are given arbitrary

---

[c]A problem in some studies of the relationship between hospital beds and physicians is that the total number of beds for a county (region, state) is used rather than the hospital bed-to-population ratio. Thus, for example, Mountin, Pennell, and Nicolay (1942b) distinguish between places with no beds, 0 to 250 beds, and over 250 beds. It is one thing, however, for a county of 100,000 to have 100 hospital beds and a county of 20,000 to have 100 hospital beds. On a ratio basis, the smaller county has a value that is five times higher.

scores of 1 to 5, with IR = 1 and GM = 5. For all counties the product-moment correlation coefficients between this scale and county median family income and percentage of urban residents are 0.51 and 0.62. The multiple correlation (R^2) is 0.41.

Both the correlation and regression coefficients between the hospital-bed and physician ratios are given in Table 10-1, for each of the county types separately for specialists and general practitioners. For ease of interpretation, regression coefficients are multiplied by 100; thus, the coefficient of 29.82 for GM-type counties means that an increase of 100 beds per 100,000 population leads, on the average, to an increase of 29.82 specialists per 100,000.

Examining the regression coefficients first, it is clear that except for the reversal between R- and AM-type counties, the regression coefficients systematically increase for specialists from IR to GM counties, from 1.04 specialists per 100,000 population with each increase of 100 in the hospital-bed ratio in isolated rural counties to 29.82 in greater metropolitan counties. The "reversal" for specialists in the AM-type counties is consistent with the earlier hypothesis, that large cities with the most specialized hospital facilities compete successfully with the suburbs (AM-type counties) in attracting specialists with hospital facilities. However, the operation of other variables besides hospital facilities in accounting for variation in the specialist ratio is the same in both county types; this is reflected by the coefficient of nondetermination $(1 - r^2)$, or residual variance, which is the same for both county types (0.815). There is no pattern in the regression coefficients for general practitioners. The interaction of county hospital facilities with income-urban level of county is clearly limited to specialists.

Table 10-1

Relationship Between Physician Ratio and Hospital-Bed Ratio, by County Type, Separately for Specialists and General Practitioners[a]

	Isolated Rural	Rural	Adjacent to Metropolitan	Lesser Metropolitan	Greater Metropolitan
Specialists					
b	1.04	11.78	6.43	18.11	29.82
r	0.24	0.43	0.43	0.59	0.83
General practitioners					
b	3.70	1.45	1.89	0.39	2.16
r	0.40	0.23	0.29	0.08	0.51

Sources: C.N. Theodore, G.E. Sutter, and E.A. Jokiel (1967).

[a]Regression coefficients are multiplied by 100.

Moreover, a comparison of the regression coefficients for the two types of physicians indicates that the (statistical) effect of hospital facilities is much greater on the specialist ratio in all county types except the Isolated Rural type. Even here, however, the effect of the hospital-bed ratio on the general practitioner ratio is quite weak in comparison to its effect on specialists in the other four county types. Therefore, although the overall effect of hospital facilities differs for specialists and general practitioners, the effect on specialists as well as the difference in the effect between specialists and general practitioners vary depending on the overall county context.

Examination of the correlation coefficients is also informative. For specialists, coefficients increase from IR- to GM-type counties, which means that the influence of other variables on the specialist ratio as reflected by the residual variance $(1 - r^2)$ systematically decreases from IR- to GM-type counties; that is, hospital facilities and the socioeconomic context of community interact in the degree of association between hospital facilities and the specialist ratio as well as in the statistical effect of hospital facilities on this ratio. As with the regression coefficients, the correlation coefficients manifest no particular pattern for general practitioners.

The hypothesis states, of course, that the effect of hospital facilities on physicians will vary depending on community income and urban levels. The classification of county type does not perfectly reflect differences in these variables, of course. (As noted previously, the R^2 for the arbitrary scale and income and percent urban is 0.41). The significance of income is clear from Figure 10-2, however. County types are scaled on the abscissa according to the *average* median family income for counties in each county type and the regression coefficients of specialist ratios on hospital-bed ratios are placed on the ordinate. Although small numbers of cases always raise questions about the magnitude of a correlation coefficient, inspection of the plots leaves little doubt about the contextual effect of county income on the relationship between hospital-bed and specialist physician ratios. The extent to which hospital-bed ratios exert an actual effect on this ratio, that is, the difference in the slope of the regression line (*b*), is clearly constrained by community wealth. It is impossible to disentangle the effects of income and urbanization because the relationship between the income and urban levels of counties is reciprocal, as noted in Chapter 3. Indeed, when income is replaced by the urban index in Figure 10-2, there is little to choose between them since $r = 0.95$.

Analysis by Regions

The above analysis was repeated separately for each of the nine census divisions. However, since there are only a few counties of some types in certain regions, certain county types were combined in six regions (e.g., GM- and

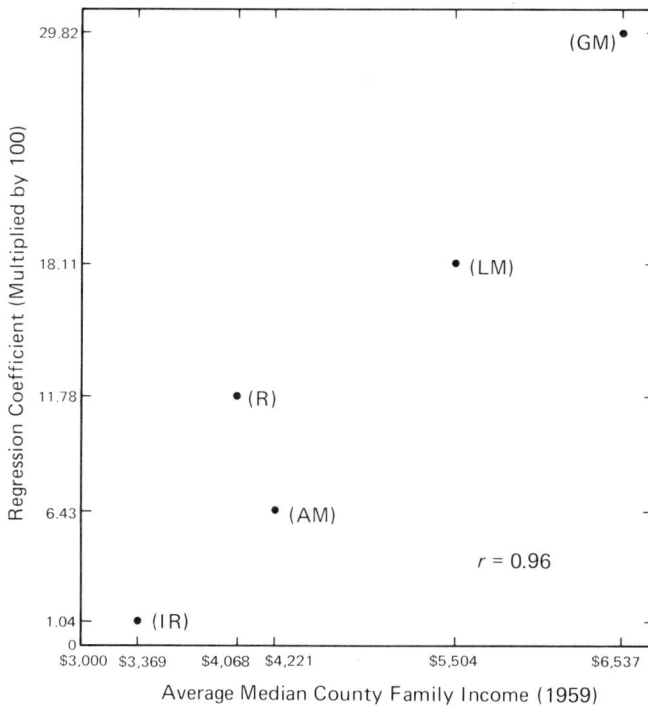

Figure 10-2. Regression Coefficient for County Specialist Ratio on Hospital-bed Ratio Plotted on Average Median Family Income for County Type

LM-types are combined for the East South Central region and R- and IR-types are combined for New England). In addition, the IR-type from the Pacific Coast was eliminated because in only 4 of 13 counties was there at least one specialist; consequently, since the other nine cases varied considerably with respect to hospital facilities, the regression coefficient is completely meaningless for this group of counties. Inspection of the scatter diagrams between community wealth and the regression coefficients of the specialist ratio on the hospital-bed ratio revealed three other unusual distributions. In New England there was an extreme case among the fifteen AM-type counties, and one extreme case each among the twenty-six GM-type and twenty-eight IR-type counties in the Middle Atlantic region. With these three counties eliminated, the correlation coefficient for all regions varied from .66 for the West North Central states to .99 for the South Atlantic states. Scatter plots for these two regions are presented in Figure 10-3.

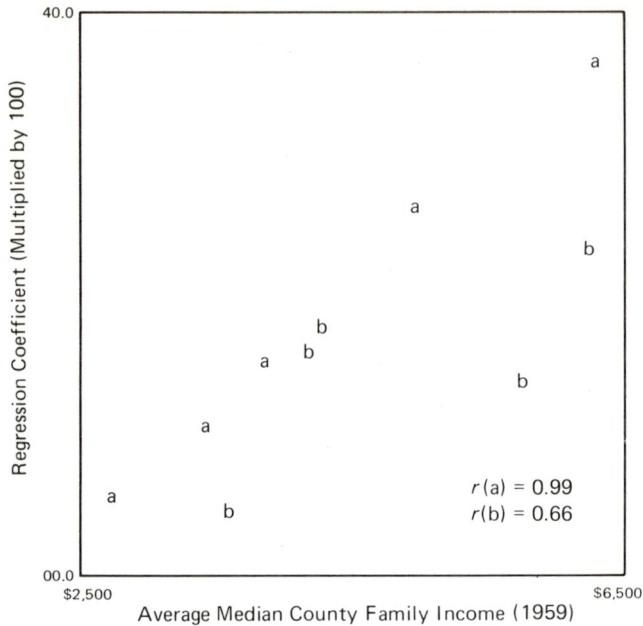

Figure 10-3. Regression Coefficients for County Specialist Ratio on Hospital-bed Ratio Plotted on Average Median Family Income for County Type for South Atlantic (a) and West North Central (b) Regions

As noted, interpretation of correlation coefficients are dubious when only a few cases are involved. In the present case, although a number of counties go into the computation in each region, the coefficients as in Figure 10-3 are based on only five cases; the relationship is between the regression coefficient of the specialist ratio on hospital-bed ratio and average county income for county types. Still, the fact that all coefficients are of substantial magnitude raises the confidence that can be placed in them. Moreover, the rank order correlation (Spearman rank correlation), which is usually a more appropriate statistic when the number of cases is small, varies from 0.64 to 1.00 between median family income and the regression of specialists on hospital beds for the nine regions.

To pursue the analysis further, regression coefficients for the physician ratio on the hospital-bed ratio were obtained for the total number of region-county type combinations and analysis identical to that in Figure 10-2 was conducted. Since there are nine regions and five county types, there are 45 possible region-county type combinations. However, as noted above, county-types were combined in six regions. This, along with the elimination of the IR-type from the Pacific Coast, gives a total of 38 region-county type combinations. The regression coefficient of each of the two physician ratios on the hospital-bed ratio are computed for these 38 units. Correlation coefficients were then computed between the regression coefficients and the income index (the average for counties within each of the 38 combinations).

In this analysis correlation coefficients of substantial magnitude would not be expected. This is so because the analysis includes county groups from different regions. Since region is also a significant factor in the distribution of physicians,[d] county groups are heterogeneous with respect to each other in matters other than overall wealth. Even so, the correlation coefficient is 0.70 for specialists and -0.10 for general practitioners. Results are similar when income is replaced with the average number of residents living in urban areas and the average professional ratio. Corresponding coefficients for the urban index are 0.76 and -0.34. For the professional ratio they are 0.78 and -0.14.[e] The constraints imposed by the general socioeconomic context of community on the relationship between hospital facilities and specialists is clear. The extent to which hospital facilities attract specialist physicians to communities depends on the nature of the communities. They are far more useful in attracting physicians in affluent and populous-dense communities with highly skilled occupational-service sectors than in less affluent, less populous-dense communities with low skilled occupational-service sectors.[f]

The Contextual Effects of Hospital Facilities

In examining the interaction of hospital facilities with the general county context on specialist physicians, analysis has been limited to the constraints of community context on hospital facilities. The obverse may also be true, however. That is, the effects of general socioeconomic aspects of community on specialists may vary depending on the level of hospital facilities that the

---

[d]The average county physician ratio varies from 115 per 100,000 population for the New England states to 59 per 100,000 for the East South Central states.

[e]Spearman rank correlations between the regression coefficients for specialists and these three variables are 0.55 (median family income) 0.42 (percent urban) and 0.51 (professional ratio).

[f]In this analysis it is assumed that the hospital-bed ratio is the independent variable and the physician ratio is the dependent variable. This is a simplifying assumption, of course, and in reality the direction of the relationships sometimes operates the other way. More probably the two are reciprocally related to some extent; hospital facilites attract specialist physicians to the community and the actions of specialists constitute a force for the establishment of additional facilities.

community is able or willing to provide. It is not likely that many communities, no matter how affluent or populous, are apt to attract large numbers of specialist physicians in the absence of hospital facilities. To explore this hypothesis the relationship is examined between county income and the physician ratio for all U.S. counties, stratified according to the hospital-bed ratio. Counties are stratified into eight groupings based on the number of hospital beds per 1,000 population: less than 1.00; 1.00-1.99; 2.00-2.99; 3.00-3.99; 4.00-4.99; 5.00-5.99; 6.00-6.99; and 7.00 and over. The regression coefficient then is computed between median family income and the two physician ratios (specialists and general practitioners) for each of the eight county groups. These coefficients are then plotted against the average hospital ratio for each of the eight groups.

Results are presented in Figure 10-4. It is clear that the relationship between community wealth and specialists varies depending on the hospital-bed ratio ($r = 0.93$). Results for the urban index and professional ratio are similar (r for the urban index is 0.95 and 0.93 for the professional ratio).

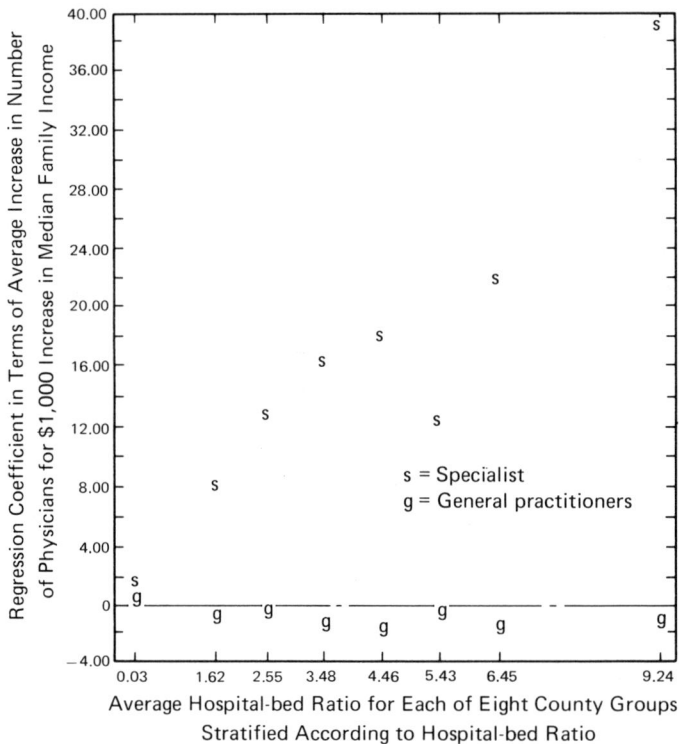

Figure 10-4. Regression Coefficients for General Practitioner and Specialty Ratios on Median Family Income Plotted on Hospital-bed Ratio for Eight County Groups, Stratified on Hospital-bed Ratio

Note, however, that the hospital-bed ratio has a very slight negative effect on general practitioners (as indicated by the very gradual negative slope). (However, the correlation coefficient is rather high, $r = -0.60$; for the urban index and professional ratio, $r = -0.83$ and -0.54.) Community contextual factors that increasingly attract specialists have an increasingly negative effect on general practitioners as the hospital-bed ratio increases. Thus, as the community hospital bed capacity increases, general community social and economic factors become increasingly important in attracting specialists to communities but appear to have the opposite effect on general practitioners. This suggests that hospitals and general practitioners are functional alternatives, at least from the standpoint of specialty practice. We turn to this hypothesis in the next chapter.

11

Specialization and Hospital Facilities: Organizational Aspects

Thus far concern has been limited to distributional aspects of physicians, and in the previous chapter with how the distribution of hospital facilities influences the distribution of physicians. In this chapter the relationship between physician manpower and hospital facilities is viewed from a different perspective, from the standpoint of health-care *organization*. The central focus remains the same; concern is still with community differences in physician manpower and how this is related to specialization. But these differences are now viewed from the standpoint of organizational patterns. A thesis of the chapter is that new organizational forms are emerging in American medicine that have a significant implication for the distributional patterns which were observed in the previous chapter.

Others have pointed to emergent forms of medical practice, such as increased group practice, prepaid capitation plans (in contrast to fee for service),[a] Health Maintenance Organizations, increased use of paramedical personnel, and other developments. The focus of this chapter, however, concerns the changing role of hospitals in the practice of medicine, especially with respect to the process through which patients reach specialists. Hospitals perform a more important role in this process today than in the past. This has occurred simultaneously with a decrease in the proportion of physicians who are general practitioners. It is possible, therefore, that both the emergence of hospitals and the decline of general practice have had an influence on the referral process. Hospitals may have replaced general practitioners to a great extent in this process.

Specialists and General Practitioners: Statistical and Functional Relationships

In considering the differences between specialists and general practitioners, differences have been observed in the relationship of the two groups to other variables, such as median family income and hospital-bed ratios. Now the relationship between the types of physicians themselves will be examined.

Statistically, there is virtually no relationship between them. For all 2,971 counties, the correlation coefficient is -0.09. The same general finding applies

---

[a]A capitation plan is one in which a physician or group of physicians are paid an annual sum for treating all patients in a specified population.

to all nine regions, with the exception of the East North Central, where the correlation coefficient is -0.30, which is still rather low. Our interest, however, is not the *statistical* relationship between the two types of physicians, but the *functional* relationship between them.

The role of the two types of physicians have not been the object of much systematic research, but some tentative conclusions would seem to be warranted based on the training and qualifications of the two types of physicians. General practitioners are trained largely to treat frequently occurring illnesses that require a minimum in diagnostic tests and therapeutic technology —for example, influenza, intestinal parasites, common colds, certain broken bones, minor burns, and the like. Specialists, on the other hand, are more qualified to treat illnesses that occur infrequently, and are often quite serious in nature; for example, heart disease, cancer, neurological lesions, urological disorders, serious allergies, and diabetes. Therefore, the functional relationship between general practitioners and specialists would appear to be one in which patients are referred to specialists by general practitioners.

It is probable that the roles of the two types of physicians in a particular community vary depending on the relative proportions of each in the community. For example, Stanley Greenhill and Harry J. Singh report that the general practitioner in rural areas is more apt than the urban general practitioner to respond to more diversified needs and to provide a wider range of services to patients; he is more apt to provide pediatric services and to perform more complicated general surgery as well as specialized surgery (Greenhill and Singh 1964, 1965). The referral rate to specialists is higher for the urban general practitioner (Greenhill and Singh 1965, p. 860). In addition, the referral rate varies in rural areas since "the roles of rural practitioner will vary in those areas where specialist care is available" (Greenhill and Singh 1964, p. 808). Thus, the role of general practitioner in the referral process would appear to depend on the presence of specialists in the community.

By the same token, the probability that specialists will receive referrals from general practitioners depends on the presence of general practitioners. (The subject has been the topic of much discussion. Without access to general practitioners, the process of reaching a specialist may be quite complicated for many patients, and for some it may be a frustrating experience indeed.) Thus, from the specialists' point of view, general practitioners can perform an important function. Indeed, general practitioners may form the base of the specialists' practice. Traditionally, specialty practice has rested on the foundation of general medical practice.

According to the results presented in previous chapters, the foundation does not appear to vary systematically very much with other characteristics of communities. But note also, looking again at Figure 7-1 (p. 103), that the regression lines for general practitioners intersects the ordinate at a higher level than the

line for all specialists.[b] Table 11-1 presents the point of intercept (the a coefficient) for the regression equation in which the two physician ratios are regressed on the hospital-bed ratio, separately for each of the five county types.
Comparison between the two types of physicians reveals that in all instances
the coefficient is much higher for general practitioners, among whom it
decreases slightly but continuously from IR-type counties to GM-type counties
(no particular pattern is evident for specialists, however). In Table 11-2 the
intercept is given for specialists and general practitioners for the 38 region-
county type combinations. Comparisons reveal that in 37 instances the intercept
is higher for general practitioners, in many instances substantially so (the coefficient for Pacific Coast rural counties is the only exception).

Since the intercept is a constant in the regression equation and for general
practitioners varies only slightly for county types (most differences in Tables
11-1 and 11-2 are quite small), results suggest that general practitioners do provide a base on which the medical community is built and that this does not vary
depending on the type of community. This is consistent with the conclusion of
the National Advisory Commission (1967, Vol. I, p. 25):

> What system of health care there is in this country is based on the 19th
> century assumption that the keystone of care is the general practitioner
> in private practice.

Table 11-1

**Point of Intercept (a) in Regression Equation for Physician Ratio on Hospital-
Bed Ratio by County Type, Separately for General Practitioners and
Specialists[a]**

	Isolated Rural	Rural	Adjacent to Metropolitan	Lesser Metropolitan	Greater Metropolitan
General practitioners	36.42	32.40	31.15	26.62	25.30
Specialists	0.66	−16.67	3.45	4.17	1.88
N	721	991	866	289	104

Sources: C. N. Theodore, G.E. Sutter, and E.A. Jokiel (1967) and U.S. Bureau of the
Census (1967).

[a]Coefficients are multiplied by 100.

---

[b]This may vary with degree of specialization, as results for states indicate (see
Figure 7-2, p. 105).

COMMUNITY, SPECIALIZATION, AND HOSPITALS

Table 11-2
Point of Intercept (a) in Regression Equation for Physician Ratio on Hospital-Bed Ratio by County Type and Region, Separately for Specialists and General Practitioners[a]

		County Type[b]				
		GM	LM	AM	R	IR
New England	Specialist	−11.3[c]		09.9	−23.9[c]	
	General Practitioner	24.5		37.7	22.9[c]	
Middle Atlantic	Specialist	−03.8	04.0	16.0	−60.8[c]	
	General Practitioner	26.0	34.1	40.6	43.0[c]	
East North Central	Specialist	09.2	−12.0	02.1	−09.9	−00.4
	General Practitioner	21.8	32.8	35.1	38.6	36.9
West North Central	Specialist	−05.7	11.9	−18.5	−45.7	02.5
	General Practitioner	16.0	20.3	36.0	40.5	25.5
South Atlantic	Specialist	16.3	−13.3	−07.3	−01.3	−01.0
	General Practitioner	17.6	19.7	25.4	29.2	28.4
East South Central	Specialist	−08.1[c]		02.6	06.9	05.4
	General Practitioner	29.3[c]		28.5	30.0	29.1
West South Central	Specialist	09.1[c]		08.1	04.8	03.4
	General Practitioner	23.7[c]		29.6	35.0	26.0
Rocky Mountain	Specialist	14.5[c]		13.0	09.6	05.0
	General Practitioner	22.2[c]		31.9	39.1	29.3
Pacific Coast	Specialist	−08.3	06.3	33.4	27.4	
	General Practitioner	29.0	29.1	42.9	27.3	

Sources: C.N. Theodore, G.E. Sutter, and E.A. Jokiel (1967) and U.S. Bureau of the Census (1967).

[a]Coefficients are multiplied by 100.

[b]GM = Greater metropolitan
LM = Lesser metropolitan
AM = Adjacent
R = Rural
IR = Isolated rural

[c]Represents combined category.

The commission also notes, however, that because of the decrease in general practitioners and increase in specialists, "the keystone has collapsed" (1967, Vol. I, p. 25).

By this I understand the commission to mean that the patients' traditional primary "point of entry" into the medical care system is (or was) the general practitioner. Traditionally in medicine, Mark G. Field notes that "the patient was . . . introduced by his GP to the health care system" (Fields 1970, p. 169). Robin F. Badgley and Samuel Wolfe have commented that "no health service, private or public, can succeed unless careful attention is paid to the doctor who provides the primary care in the community. All other decisions depend on what he decides when the patient is first seen." (Badgley and Wolfe 1967, p. 134.) Thus, in the words of Field, "the allocative [referral] functions usually played by a general practitioner are a necessary complement to specialization . . . . The patient . . . needs . . . a helping hand in finding the appropriate portal into the medical system (that is, a generalist in the community). . . ." (Field 1970, pp. 170, 172). Consequently, with the decline of general practitioners, the foundation by which patients are able to get from generalist to specialist and from specialist to specialist (as well as to receive that care which the general practitioner is qualified to give) will gradually disappear. "With the absolute and proportional decline of general practice in the community, . . . the patient has lost his portal entry into the medical system" (Field 1970, p. 169). It is possible, however, that this particular system of medical care may be giving way to another system; other agents may be replacing general practitioners in the referral functions traditionally performed by general practitioners. While the traditional base of medical practice may be disappearing, another base may be emerging.

The Organizational Perspective

Before considering this question in more detail, the question of the relationship between general practitioners and specialists will be explored from an organizational perspective. Although the focus of this book is the distribution of physicians, (emerging) organizational trends should not be divorced from the issue. Moreover, as is argued in Chapter 16, it is in terms of organizational changes that the distributional problem is most likely to be alleviated.

One of the truisms of sociology is that as social systems and social institutions become increasingly differentiated—where individual roles become quite specialized, there is a corresponding need for some mechanism to perform integrative functions. Different mechanisms exist in different types of institutions. In many manufacturing plants where individual workers are responsible for performing a very small (but repetitive) operation in the overall scheme of operations, the assembly line is a regulatory or integrative force; the pace of the "belt" determines when the worker does what he does. In other institutions where regulation of overall operations is not built into the work flow itself, supervision of subordinates by superiors who understand the way all the parts fit together is the primary method of integration. In systems such as hospitals, universities, and other organizations in which a large proportion of the activity involves the processing of persons, scheduling is important. And also in organizations such as universities and hospitals where a large proportion of the employees are professionally and technically trained, workers are expected to be reliable and to be motivated by their technical knowledge of what needs to be done; control and integration is based more than in other systems on the motivation, attitudes and knowledge of the workers themselves.

With the increase in specialization, the question arises as to whether the sociological truism applies to physicians. There are some reasons to expect that it does not. Physicians do not themselves constitute an organization. Even at the local community level, each physician usually has his own individual practice, and while physicians may share common hospital facilities, cooperate as members of the hospital staff, and belong to the same local, state, and national medical societies, individual practices are generally not coordinated with reference to each other in a purposive way. Each physician tends to treat and be medically committed to particular patients from the community, and the particular patients differ from physician to physician. Physicians do not generally view the entire community as the patient and their commitment tends not to be to the community as a whole. And what one physician does in reference to his patients may be unrelated to what other physicians do. In short, the actions of physicians tend not to be coordinated with reference to each other, except for such things as when they may use certain hospital facilities.

The picture is overdrawn to a certain extent. Physicians are probably integrated into a network of relationships—"the colleague network"—at the local community level to a greater extent than is commonly recognized (Friedson 1963). This network refers to the informal relationships that exist among physicians in community settings. While such relationships have not been the object of extensive systematic study, some fragmentary and suggestive evidence does exist. (See Friedson 1963; Hall 1946, 1948; and Shortell 1973, 1974.)

Apparently, cooperative arrangements develop between local physicians so that one's practice is covered by colleagues who can be trusted not to steal his patients; norms regulating fee charges tend to develop; referral systems emerge, with physicians referring patients only to certain colleagues and usually to physicians whose status in the network is higher than their own; recruitment is controlled to some degree through the referral process (e.g., a new physician who does not become part of the informal network may fail to receive referrals from established physicians—at least referrals with the ability to pay); new physicians are sometimes sponsored by older members of the network, and when in need a new member is expected to turn to his sponsor for advice. The network appears to extend to hospitals, and may be most powerful in communities where hospitals exist. Access to hospital facilities and hence access to patients may depend upon entrance into the informal network. In communities with several hospitals, hospitals and patients no less than physicians may be tied to different physician networks.

Nevertheless, the picture of an *aggregate* (not an organization) of independent practitioners is not altogether inaccurate. Certainly the view of physicians as independent and autonomous is more valid than the picture of physicians as members of organizations in which mechanisms of integration and coordination are deliberately created; the medical industry is very much a "cottage industry." It is probable, however, that traditionally there has been a mechanism of integration, though not one that has been deliberately created.

This mechanism is the network of referrals. I am not talking about the lay referral system in which individuals are referred to physicians by relatives, friends and by the physician's general reputation in the community (cf. Friedson 1960). Such referrals are probably limited to general practitioners and to the generalists among the specialists. My concern here is how patients get to the more specialized physicians—e.g., urologists, orthopedists, radiologists, cancer specialists, neurologists, allergists, and specialized surgeons. In many instances the patient does not know where to go except to the more general physician; only after examinations and tests have been made by a generalist is the need for more specialized treatment established. Moreover, many specialists will not see patients unless they have been referred to them by other physicians (they will not take "walk-ins"), and this usually means referrals from physicians in more general practice. According to this view, then, the network of referrals provides for a degree of coordination among physicians: generalists depend on specialists to whom they can send patients for tests, examinations and treatments that are beyond their competence to perform, while the specialists depend on the more generalized physicians for the source of their patients.

According to this view, before specialists exist in a community generalists must also exist. In addition, since limited specialists (e.g., neurosurgeons) are more specialized than general specialists (e.g., internists), the referral process would typically go from the latter to the former. Consequently, whereas the presence of general specialists in a community depends on the presence of generalists, the presence of limited specialists depends on the presence of general specialists as well as general practitioners. Medical specialization is analogous to a pyramid, with the most general skills represented at the base and the more limited specialists at the apex. The ability of communities to attract and keep specialists will depend on how well the base below the specialists' level has been laid.

Although data are not available on the full range of medical specialties for all counties in the United States to test this conception, data are available for 36 specialties for 87 counties that compose the region of the Tennessee

Mid-South Regional Medical Program (TMS/RMP). In 1966 TMS/RMP conducted a survey of physicians by specialty in this region. I have classified physicians into generalists, general specialists, and limited specialists, as in previous analysis. Counties are classified into three categories, as follows: (1) counties with all three types of physicians; (2) counties with at least one general practitioner and one general specialist, but no limited specialist; and (3) counties with only general practitioners. The hypothesis is that all counties can be classified in one of these categories. For example, there would be no county with a limited specialist but no generalist or general specialist. Eighty-three of the eighty-seven counties could be placed in one of the three county types. This supports the hypothesis that certain types of physicians constitute a support base for other types of physicians. Most general physicians do not require the support of other types of physicians; they can function in communities in which specialists do not exist. The next most general physicians—general specialists— exist in communities only if there are general practitioners. And the most specialized physicians exist only in communities that have both general practitioners and general specialists. This suggests that general practitioners provide a support base on which general and limited specialists are overlaid.

But this relationship is to be viewed within the broader context of the community. This is seen in Table 11-3. Since counties vary widely with respect to the number of limited specialists, category (3) above is divided into five separate groups. Except for the separation of counties which have 1 to 2 limited specialists and 3 to 6 limited specialists, points of separation for the number of limited specialists conform to clear-cut points of separation in the distribution (e.g., there were no counties that have 14 to 29 specialists, so that counties with 8 to 13 specialists are distinguished from those with 30 to 44 specialists). The average population (1970) as well as the average family income (1969) for counties in each group are reported.[c] The relationships of physician mix to county income and size of county population are clear. Counties with only general practitioners have the lowest average population and median family income. Next lowest is the group that has only general practitioners and general specialists, with counties having limited specialists ranking highest but rank within this group depending on the number of specialists. The results qualify the earlier conclusion about the relationships between income and urban levels of counties and medical specialization. The relationships do exist, but different compositions of physicians require different types of support within the medical

---

[c]I noted earlier (pp. 31) that the use of density (population per square mile) is problematical when communities differ in the physical area they cover. This is the reason for using percent urban residents rather than density (or total population) in the analysis. In the case of Tennessee Mid-South, there is very little variation between counties in square miles; the product-moment correlation between total population and population per square mile is 0.92. Consequently, population density and total population are substitutable. In the present instance, we report figures for the total population.

Table 11-3

Average County Population and Median Family Income for Different Physician Composition for the 87 Counties in the Tennessee Mid-South Region

Physician Composition[a]	Average Population[b]	Average Median Family Income[c]
General practitioners only (N = 34)[d]	11,554	5,402
General practitioners plus at least one general specialist (N = 17)	16,425	5,816
General practitioners and general specialists plus 1-2 limited specialists (N = 15)[e]	27,098	6,430
General practitioners and general specialists plus 3-6 limited specialists (N = 9)	35,690	6,940
General practitioners and general specialists plus 8-13 limited specialists (N = 4)	56,818	7,442
General practitioners and general specialists plus 30-44 limited specialists (N = 5)	75,426	7,628
General practitioners and general specialists plus 144-366 limited specialists (N = 3)	326,177	8,759

[a]Source: Tennessee Mid-South Regional Medical Program, "Professional Survey of Physicians," 1966, Appendix A. Generalized specialists includes general surgeons, pediatricians, obstetricians, gynecologists, and internists. Limited specialists include all other specialists.

[b]U.S. Bureau of the Census, (1973a).

[c]U.S. Bureau of the Census (1973a).

[d]Includes two counties with no general practitioner but one generalized specialist (general surgeon and obstetrician-gynecologist).

[e]Includes two counties with no generalized specialists.

sector. Limited specialists require more than certain general economic and urban conditions; they also require the presence of less specialized physicians who will treat patients not requiring more specialized medical skills and who will refer to appropriate specialists those patients needing types of care that only limited specialists are able to provide. And general specialists (in 32 of 34 counties) require the presence of general practitioners to treat a wide range of problems that do not require the skills of either general or limited specialists. Although the general economic context and population base of a community impose constraints on the range of medical services available in a community, the presence of physicians with more general skills also places constraints on the recruitment of physicians higher on the scale of specialization.

In light of earlier findings, this view suggests that the base of a referral system (general practitioners) exists in most types of counties in the United States (although it is shrinking), but many of the specialists to whom patients can be referred by general practitioners do not exist. Poor, rural communities tend not to have specialist services available to them. They are almost totally dependent on primary care providers, if available at all, when specialized care is needed. A different kind of problem may exist in the more affluent, urban areas. In these settings the primary danger may be that the patient does not receive the continuity of care that contact with primary care physicians may provide; a patient may see many specialists, but there is no physician with an overall picture of the patients' medical status to provide a general guide to care.

When viewed from this perspective, results indicate several conclusions about the future. General practitioners are declining and will probably continue to do so. The effect of this on economically depressed areas will be to reduce medical manpower further, and the effect in more affluent, urban counties will be to reduce the strength of the referral network on which specialist care has been based. In economically depressed and sparsely populated areas less primary care will be available and the opportunity for people to get into a referral network will be diminished even more—because of the presence of few specialists as well as the reduction in general practitioners. For the more affluent populous areas the consequence will be relatively less primary care than is now the case and a strain on the referral system. To an increasing extent, a larger proportion of the population will have no central "point of entry" into the referral network, and continuity of care will become an even greater problem than it is now.[d]

The general problem is common for systems undergoing increases in the level of differentiation. In many systems, integrative functions are delegated,

---

[d]Data concerning the status of the suburbs are lacking but the following would appear to be consistent with earlier results. Since the suburbs are attracting generalists from the inner city, they would seem to be most able to provide community members with a sufficient level of general services and specialty services. Patients may be referred to the more limited specialists in nearby cities, since limited specialists appear not to have moved to the suburbs to the same extent as the more general physicians. Hence, rural, low-income areas have a deficit of overall medical manpower, but the manpower they do have is limited largely to general and family practitioners; the inner cities have a larger supply of the very specialized physicians but a deficiency of physicians with general and primary care skills; and in the suburbs physicians with general skills appear to be growing faster than those with limited highly specialized skills, although there is a good supply of the latter available in nearby cities.

sometimes to lower echelon personnel.[e] Problems of medical care are compounded, however, by the fact that the physician role of performing coordinative functions in medicine is disappearing. Mark Field observes, *"there is no one with medical professional training who stands below the general practitioner.* If one reaches below the GP to scoop someone with medical training who could fit into the physician's shoes, there is, in truth, no one with these qualifications. The result is that the functions of the general practitioner are often not being performed by a medical person; or that someone else, without appropriate professional qualifications, steps into that role and performs like a generalist. This is what, to some degree, is taking place in the American medical system." (Field 1970, p. 167; author's emphasis).

In organizational terms, then, the system of health care delivery has become increasingly complex—there are more kinds of physicians to go to for different ailments and patients receive a greater variety of services from more different types of specialists in different settings. What was formerly done by the general practitioner in one setting is now done by many providers in different settings. Whereas the general practitioner was previously able to coordinate all (or nearly all) the services a patient received, this is no longer the case. That role has increasingly become the *patient's* responsibility. James D. Thompson (1973, p. 33) states:

> What we now refer to as a "Health-Care-Delivery System" involves private practitioners (sometimes in series), clinics, laboratories, nurses, technicians, dietitians, aides and orderlies, therapists of various sorts, accountants, third-party-payers, and computer specialists—to say nothing of patients and their families. Unless my experiences have been very unusual, those components operate as reasonably competent components but rather incompetently as elements in a larger system. To the extent that there is coordination among them, it is the patient or patient-representative who must bring it about. It appears to me that each component in his complicated system is telling the client that he/she must worry about the articulation—that it is too complicated for the health care delivery system to handle.

Consequently, some persons view the demise of the general practitioner as

---

[e]The evolution of coordinative hospital roles to nurses is generally well known and, in many respects, actually accepted by physicians, hospital administrators and nurses themselves. For example, some authors even define the nurse role as coordinative (Alfano 1970, p. 2117; Mauksch 1965). This role is not accepted by all health professionals; it has been a source of some controversy, complaints, and criticisms. See Jerome P. Lysault (1970), and Luther Christman and Richard C. Jellinek (1967).

a cause for alarm. It represents the collapse of the medical system, with much fragmented care but with little or no coordination, except that which the patient gives to it. Such a view suggests that medical care in the United States is highly disorganized and, indeed, bordering on chaos.

Although the picture may be overdrawn, the burden being assumed by the individual patient *is* heavy, and is undoubtedly the source of much public frustration with medicine, as some of the above comments would suggest. Public pressure will probably not permit the process to continue, and certainly resistance can be expected if it does. It is probable, to quote from Thompson again, "that we are going to have to learn to absorb [the complexity of health care delivery] into the system [itself], rather than pushing it off onto the client" (Thompson 1973, p. 333). But is the general practitioner the only element (or even the best element) of the system in which such complexity is to be absorbed? The fact that general practitioners performed such a role in the past is not, by that fact alone, grounds for assuming that they represent the only or best mechanism for performing this function today and in the future. Moreover, will there be enough of them to perform such a role in the future? Given the current trends it is not likely. I suggest that the history of medicine shows that the allocative and coordinative roles in specialized care have shifted from general practitioners to patients and that these roles are now shifting to other elements of the delivery system. For many patients, the referral process and the central point of entry into the medical system may be changing.

Field notes, for example, that "the modern hospital has become, in the last 50 years, the center of the medical world. Conceptually, furthermore, the process of specialization that has taken place in the medical profession may also be seen if the hospital is visualized as a kind of 'collective physician.'" (Field 1970, p. 164). The functions performed by this "collective physician" may include the referral functions previously performed by the general practitioner as well as the functions of the many specialists who are on the hospital staff. Indeed, given the decrease in physicians who perform coordinative functions of patient care, it would not be surprising to find that this is the case. Accordingly, we would expect that hospital emergency service and outpatient clinics (as well as other clinics, such as neighborhood health centers) will become primary points of entry into the medical world for an increasing proportion of the population. This seems to have already begun. For example, between 1947 and 1966 the average number of outpatient visits per community hospital in the United States increased by 233 percent (roughly 10 percent per year, on the average), whereas the number of inpatient admissions increased by only 69 percent (American Hospital Association 1967, p. 445). There is no way to know if the number of outpatient hospital visits represents a greater proportion of all physician visits over this period. It is doubtful, however, if the average physician's daily patient load has more than doubled during this time. In any case, relative to the inpatient service, the role of hospitals in ambulatory care has increased. It is clear that more outpatient treatment is being provided in hospital settings. And if this continues, medicine in the future will be practiced increasingly in such settings. "The institutionalization of medical care resulting from the shifting of the locus of medical services to the hospital (the medical supermarket) and the increase in specialty practices will continue" (Field 1970, p. 174). This is reflected in the increase in physicians who are full-time hospital staff. Excluding all residents and interns, the number of physicians employed full time in hospitals increased by 64 percent between 1963 and 1971 in comparison to a 14 percent increase for physicians in office-based practice (Roback 1972, p. 64; Theodore and Sutter 1966, p. 38).[f] Obviously if this trend continues, medicine in the future will be practiced increasingly in hospital settings. Consequently hospitals will probably become increasingly important in the referral process to specialists.

General Practitioners, Hospitals, and the Referral Process

Note that the above trends have occurred simultaneously with a decrease both in the relative proportion of physicians who are general practitioners as well as their absolute number (for example, general practitioners decreased from 67,518 in 1963 to 52,073 in 1971) (Roback 1972, p. 64; Theodore and Sutter 1966, p. 38). Now if the referral process is an important factor in specialty practice and if this function is performed by both physicians in hospitals and general practitioners outside hospitals, certain specific relationships would be expected. If hospitals are replacing general practitioners in the referral process, it would be expected that the county hospital-bed ratio would be less important in attracting and keeping specialists in counties where the general practitioner ratio is high than where it is low. Specifically, in counties where the general practitioner ratio is high, a lower regression coefficient of the specialist ratio on the hospital-bed ratio would be expected than in counties where the general practitioner ratio is low.

To test this hypothesis, counties are divided into six groupings depending on the number of general practitioners per 100,000 population (with the number of counties in parenthesis): less than 20 (425); 20-29 (652); 30-39 (781); 40-49 (562); 50-59 (294); and 60 and above (257). For each grouping, the regression coefficient of the specialist ratio on the hospital-bed ratio is computed. If the reasoning is correct—that hospitals are functional alternatives or equivalents to general practitioners in the referral process to specialists, the

---

[f]Group practice is also growing at a rapid rate (McNamara and Todd 1970; Paxton 1969). This underscores the thesis that medical care will be provided in organizational settings with increasing frequency in the future.

regression coefficient would be higher for counties in which the general practitioner ratio is low than where it is high. Therefore, regression coefficients are plotted on the average general practitioner ratio for each of the above six groups in Figure 11-1 (e.g., the average general practitioner ratio for counties with less than 20 general practitioners per 100,000 is 10.58 per 100,000). The coefficients are multiplied by 100. Results are clear: The regression coefficient consistently decreases as the general practitioner ratio increases, except for counties with the highest ratio for general practitioners. The ability of hospital facilities to attract specialists to a community increases as the supply of general practitioners decreases.

It was noted, of course, that the regression of specialists on hospital beds also varies depending on social and economic characteristics of counties. Therefore, results in Figure 11-1 could conceivably be due to the effects of these characteristics. This is not likely, however, because the correlations between the general practitioner ratio and median income and percent urban are so low

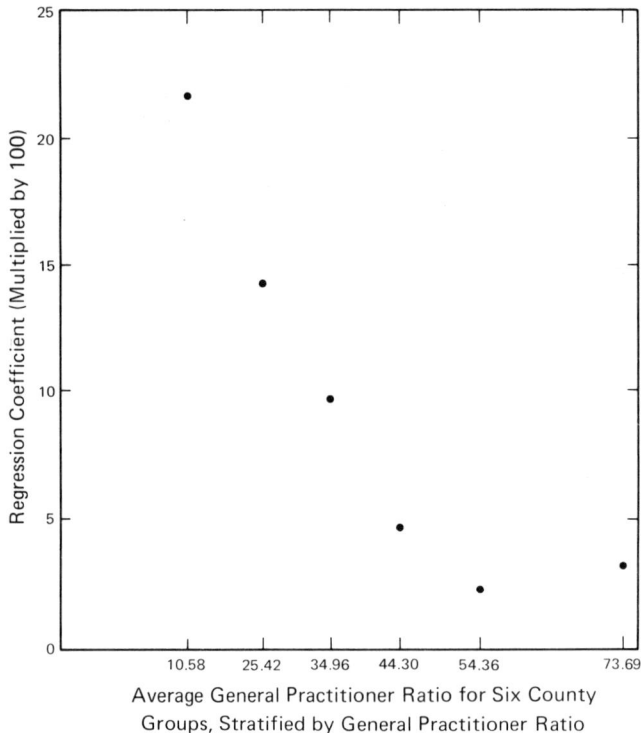

Figure 11-1. Regression Coefficient for Specialist Ratio on Hospital-Bed Ratio Plotted on General Practitioner Ratio for Six County Groups

(0.06 and -0.02). This is confirmed by the results in Table 11-4. In this table regression coefficients for the specialist ratio on the hospital-bed ratio (multiplied by 100) are reported by level of general practitioner ratio for different county types. Because the number of counties with more than 60 general practitioners per 100,000 is so low for some county types, these counties are combined with counties in the 50 to 59 range. Also, because of the relatively few counties in the two metropolitan categories, Lesser Metropolitan and Greater Metropolitan are combined into a single metropolitan category.

Inspection indicates that the effect of hospital facilities on specialists is inversely related to county general practitioner ratio in all four county types. In all but one comparison between adjacent categories (between 30-39 and 40-49 general practitioners per 100,000 among metropolitan counties) the regression coefficient is highest for the category with the smallest general practitioner ratio. In all there are 40 comparisons between categories within county types; in 39 instances the category with the highest general practitioner ratio has the lowest regression coefficient. Hospital facilities have a greater effect on the supply of community specialists when the supply of general practitioners is low than when it is high. This of course is consistent with the hypothesis that hospitals and general practitioners are functional substitutes insofar as the referral process to specialist care is concerned.

Table 11-4

Regression Coefficient of Specialist Ratio on Hospital-Bed Ratio, by County Type and County General Practitioner Ratio[a]

County Type	*General Practitioner Ratio*				
	Less Than 20	*20-29*	*30-39*	*40-49*	*50 and Above*
Metropolitan	26.5 (55)[b]	20.1 (161)	16.8 (129)	17.3 (30)	8.2 (8)
Adjacent to metropolitan	16.3 (105)	10.2 (173)	9.5 (242)	4.3 (192)	0.9 (154)
Rural	41.8 (64)	18.3 (203)	8.6 (269)	4.5 (234)	2.8 (221)
Isolated rural	4.9 (191)	3.6 (115)	1.5 (141)	0.9 (106)	1.5 (168)

Sources: C. N. Theodore, G.E. Sutter, and E.A. Jokiel (1967) and U.S. Bureau of the Census (1967).

[a]Coefficients are multiplied by 100.

[b]Figure in parentheses is number of counties.

Note also, however, that the interaction between county type and hospital facilities on the specialist ratio is independent of the county general practitioner ratio. This can be seen by observing the variation in the coefficients within columns, so that the general practitioner ratio is held constant. In all but one instance the highest coefficient is for Metropolitan counties and in all instances the lowest coefficient is for Isolated Rural counties. The reversal between the Adjacent to Metropolitan and Rural counties that was noticed in the previous chapter remains, and is probably a reflection of the effects of suburbanization.

Conclusion

Two major historical trends in medicine are the decline in general practice and the increase in specialists' dependence on hospitals. I suggest that there are important functional relationships between the two trends, since general practitioners and hospitals provide a referral mechanism for specialist treatment. Results have been presented that are consistent with this hypothesis. Since specialization will probably increase and, hence, tend to result in an increased concentration of physicians in fewer communities, the problem of how citizens in communities with low physician manpower can get referred to specialists may become more severe in the future. Results of this chapter suggest that the use of hospitals may provide (*is* providing) a focal point through which such referrals can be (and are) processed. A proposal designed to reduce inequities in medical care that incorporates this role of hospitals is presented in Chapter 16.

Part III

Programs of Action

12 Changing the Characteristics of Physicians

The basic problem in changing the maldistribution of physicians is, of course, to provide more medical services for communities where medical manpower and services are in short supply. A number of programs have been recommended for doing this, and some have been and are currently being implemented. In this and the next four chapters several of them are examined in light of the analysis and interpretations presented in Part I and Part II. They are also examined in light of some general principles about policy programs and social problems.

Before any program is successful in dealing with a social problem, two general steps are essential. First, a cause of the problem must be identified. Second, a strategy of administrative or political action must be developed that will result in a change in the causal condition; for example, too few physicians might be considered a cause of the uneven distribution of physicians, and political or administrative action might then be designed to encourage or coerce medical schools to produce more graduates. In light of these two steps, programs may be unsuccessful for two general reasons.

First, programs may be designed to influence a condition, X, that is not really a cause of the problem. Condition X may merely be something that politicians, administrators, or the general public believe is a cause of the problem. In some instances evidence may actually indicate that X is statistically associated with the problem. However, the condition X may be related to the problem only because X and the problem are both causally related to some more general factor(s). Consequently, programs that change X do not alleviate the problem because the causes of both X and the problem itself have not been changed. Thus, the first reason programs designed to cope with social problems may fail is because they are based simply on false beliefs about the causes of the problem or because they are based on an erroneous causal interpretation of the evidence.

Second, programs may be designed to change a true cause of the problem, but the cause may be a condition that cannot be changed through political and administrative action. Results have indicated, for example, that the percentage of urban residents in counties is a causal factor in the maldistribution of physicians. It is not likely, however, that the concentration of the population can be changed greatly through administrative actions. Therefore, to identify a causal condition of a problem does not *in itself* indicate that programs should be developed to make changes in that condition. At the same time, studies which identify causes that cannot be changed through administrative or political action do yield information that can be used in policy planning. Results of such studies bear on policy planning in at least three ways. First, they may rule out of consideration programs that are not feasible or practical. Second, they direct us to continue the search for "policy variables"—that is, causal conditions that may be changed through political and administrative planning. Third, to the extent that such variables are identified, knowledge of causal conditions that cannot be changed should influence the shape of programs directed to policy variables. Specifically, programs that are designed to manipulate and change one causal condition must be developed and implemented within the constraints imposed by other conditions.

Unfortunately, the distinction between policy variables and constraints is not always clear. First, conditions that from one perspective are constraints, may be from another perspective conditions that can be changed through public policy. For example, a free society such as we have in the United States may be considered an important cause of the maldistribution problem. If physicians were not free to locate their practices where they wish and were constrained instead to locate in underserved areas according to the judgments of politicians, administrators, or others, physicians would not be distributed as unevenly as they are now. Consequently, the existing societal value system that gives physicians (and others) the right to locate where they choose is a constraint on programs that are designed to alleviate the problem; it is a constraint within which programs that have other causal conditions as their focus must be developed and implemented. From another perspective, however, one may view the freedom of physicians to work and live where they choose as a policy variable. In this case, laws might be passed which restrict physicians' freedom of movement. The societal value system and character of a free society might change also, since such a law would probably not be limited in application to physicians. In any case, a value system that gives freedom to physicians to locate where they choose imposes constraints on programs that would not exist if the value system were different. Consequently, programs designed to modify the distribution of physicians would be different in a society where individuals have maximum freedom to live and work where they choose than in societies where serious limitations are placed on this freedom. Hence, whether this freedom is viewed as a policy variable or as a constraint will influence the shape of programs designed to deal with the problem.

Also, a condition may be both a policy variable and a constraint, as when a condition can be changed but only partially so. In this case it may be something that planners attempt to change but recognize that few positive results may be expected. Effective planners will also recognize, however, that the condition is a constraint within which programs, designed to change other causal conditions, are to be developed. For example, specialization may be considered a cause of the maldistribution of physicians. Consequently, if medical schools attempt to train physicians so that more are oriented to general and family practice, physicians might not be so unevenly distributed in the population. But in light of the technological and knowledge base for specialization, only a small change in the proportion of general and family practitioners might be expected. Programs designed to change other conditions that influence the distribution of physicians should then be shaped in light of the constraints imposed by specialization.

Although the distinction between policy variables and constraining conditions is not always precise, it is essential that before programs can successfully alleviate the maldistribution of physicians they must identify a cause (or causes) of the problem and establish to what extent the cause is subject to change through public policy. In this and the next four chapters, programs will be examined with this in mind.

All programs that have been recommended for dealing with the maldistribution of physicians are based on assumptions (implicitly or explicitly) as to the cause of the problem. Causes may be classified into five categories, depending on where the cause of the problem is assumed to be: individual characteristics of physicians; supply of physician manpower and the demand for medical care; the location of training institutions; medical characteristics of communities; or organizational aspects of medicine. In this chapter programs that focus on characteristics of individual physicians are examined.

If it can be shown that physicians with certain characteristics are more apt to locate in underserved areas than physicians with other characteristics, programs might be designed to produce physicians with the desired characteristics. For example, results of this study have shown that physicians from low-income and rural county backgrounds and those entering general and family practice are more apt to locate in underserved areas than are physicians who come from high-income and urban counties, and who enter specialties. An implication, therefore, is that recruiting more medical students from low-income, rural areas and training more general and family practitioners would result in an increase in the supply of physicians in low-income, rural areas. Indeed, the Comprehensive Health Manpower Training Act of 1971 allows financial aid to medical schools for developing special programs in these two areas (see Carter et al. 1974). In this chapter the probable consequences of these two programs for the maldistribution problem are examined.

Training More Generalists

The decline in general and family physicians has been viewed with alarm by many persons, both in and outside the field of medicine, for a number of years. Some claim, and others imply, that the maldistribution of physicians is created largely by specialization and the emphasis given to specialty careers in medical schools (cf. Fein 1967). Therefore, according to this argument, the training of more general and family practitioners would result in more physicians for underserved communities. The conclusion would seem consistent with the results in Chapter 7. There are serious limitations of this policy, however.

First, it was noted in Chapter 9 that the suburbanization process may have influenced the location patterns of general and family practitioners more than limited specialists. Hence, training more general and family practitioners, as well as general specialists typically associated with primary care (internists, pediatricians, and obstetrician-gynecologists), might further increase the supply of physicians for the suburbs at the expense of the inner cities. But the effect on the supply of physicians in rural and low-income counties might be severely limited as well. This is because the wealthy, more urban counties produce so many more physicians than the poor, rural counties. The problem may be seen by examining the relationship between specialization and income of county of practice for the class of 1960 with income of county of origin controlled.

In Chapter 7 it was reported that the Gamma coefficient between specialization and income of county of practice was 0.16 (see Table 7-1). Since income for physician's county of origin is also related to the income for his county of practice ($r = 0.39$; see p. 64), it is theoretically possible that level of specialization and income of county of practice are related only because both are related to income of county of origin. The relationship between specialization and income for county of practice may exist only because each is caused by a common variable—income level of county of origin.

To investigate this possibility, the relationship between income of county of practice and specialization is examined for physicians from different origins, as in Table 12-1. Since variation in income of county of origin is restricted to within income intervals, the effects of income of origin are "controlled" (or at least they are minimized) within intervals. For each interval a Gamma is computed between income of county of practice and specialization.[a] In addition, the average income of counties of practice is given for each interval, by specialty.

If specialization has no effect on where physicians locate their practice independent of the influence of county of origin, the Partial Gamma would be zero. However, the Partial Gamma is 0.11, which is only slightly less than the Gamma in which income of county of origin was not controlled (0.16). Results thus indicate that training a higher proportion of generalists would help to increase the supply of physicians in lower income counties.

Such influence would be most limited, however. In the first place, as noted, the Partial Gamma with income for county of origin controlled is less than the original Gamma. Hence, part of the relationship observed earlier, and possibly in other studies, between specialization and type of community practice setting

---

[a]The points of separation for income of counties of practice for computing Gammas are less than $4,000, $4,000-$4,999, $5,000-$5,999, $6,000-$6,999, and $7,000 and over.

Table 12-1

Average Median Family Income of County of Practice by Income of County of Origin and Specialty, and Gammas Between Median Family Income of County of Practice and Specialization

Median Family Income of County of Origin	Generalists	General Specialists	Limited Specialists	Gamma
$7,000 and over	$6,865 (N=23)	$6,611 (N=86)	$6,485 (N=172)	−0.05
$6,000-$6,999	$6,123 (N=100)	$6,362 (N=211)	$6,361 (N=429)	0.03[a]
$5,000-$5,999	$5,730 (N=76)	$6,188 (N=239)	$6,304 (N=403)	0.17[b]
$4,000-$4,999	$5,080 (N=47)	$5,792 (N=89)	$5,865 (N=156)	0.26[b]
$3,000-$3,999	$4,851 (N=34)	$5,388 (N=49)	$5,481 (N=71)	0.23[b]
Less than $3,000	$4,009 (N=31)	$4,838 (N=27)	$5,360 (N=38)	0.48[b]

Partial Gamma = 0.11

Sources: AAMC Longitudinal Study and U.S. Bureau of the Census (1967).

[a]$P = 0.03$, based on chi-square, 10 df.

[b]$P \leq .001$, based on chi-square, 10 df.

is due to the fact that both specialization and type of practice setting are related to type of community in which physicians were reared. But more important, the type of physician most apt to be effected comes from low-income counties; for example, the strongest effect of specialization is for physicians from counties with less than $3,000 annual median family income, for whom the Gamma is 0.48. Unfortunately, only 4.2 percent of all graduates in the class of 1960 are from this group of counties. In contrast, the bulk of physicians come from high-income counties (45.1 percent come from counties in which income was $6,000 and above), and for this group of physicians the effect of specialization on location is virtually nil (Gammas = -0.05 and 0.03). A substantial proportion of all three groups of physicians from these counties practice in the same (or similar) counties and there are no significant differences between the three groups. Results for urban level of county are similar. Whereas the overall Gamma between specialization and urban level of county of practice is 0.25, it is only 0.12 for physicians who were reared in counties with at least 90 percent urban residents.[b] Consequently, a greater emphasis in training physicians with general rather than specialized skills and orientations would, at least on the basis of these results, have only a limited impact on the supply of physicians in low-income, rural counties. This is because the type of physician whose choice of practice setting is most apt to be influenced by his level of specialization (that is, the physician from low-income, rural areas), constitutes such a small proportion of all physicians.

Recruiting Students from Low-Income, Rural Counties

The comprehensive Health Manpower Training Act of 1971 encourages medical schools to recruit students on the basis of individual characteristics that are believed to lead individuals to practice in underserved areas. The act authorizes financial aid to medical schools to

> establish and operate projects designed to identify, and increase admission to and enrollment in schools of medicine . . . of individuals whose background and interest make it reasonable to assume that they will engage in the practice of their profession in rural and other areas having a severe shortage of [physicians].

Since results have shown that physicians from low-income, rural counties are far more apt than physicians of different backgrounds to practice in low-income, rural counties, it is reasonable to assume that recruiting more students from these areas would result in these settings getting a higher proportion of medical school graduates than they do now.[c] Such a program in itself, however, would have very limited results.

The problem can be seen from the results of Chapter 8, in which the relationship between county of origin and county of practice was examined with specialization controlled (that is, the relationship was examined separately for each of the three physician groups—see Table 8-4 and Figure 8-1). The difference between that analysis and the one on which Table 12-1 is based is to be noted. The analysis for Table 12-1 views income of county of origin as antecedant to both the physician's decision to specialize and the selection of his county

---

[b]Gammas for each of three groups are as follows: less than 70% urban (Gamma = 0.35); 70.0%-89.9% (Gamma = 0.23) and 90.0% and more (Gamma = 0.12).

[c]A study of the regional distribution of physicians in England concludes that a region with a shortage of physicians could increase its supply of physicians by recruiting larger numbers of students from families in the region (Last 1967, p. 799).

of practice. It was controlled to see if the relationship between specialization and income for county of practice was the result of these two variables being caused by the same antecedant condition. The relationships between the three variables were viewed differently in Chapter 8; in that case, specialization was viewed as an intervening variable between income of county of origin and county of practice. It was controlled to see if it influenced the tendency of physicians to practice in settings similar to the ones in which they were reared. Results showed that specialization is indeed an important variable; it is related both to income of county of origin and of practice and its control modifies the strength of the relationship between these two variables. The strength of the relationship is inversely related to level of specialization (see Table 8-4 and Figure 8-1). However, for none of the three groups does the correlation and regression coefficients reduce to zero; all r's and b's are substantially greater than 0.00 for both county income and urbanization. This means that the effects of county of origin on selection of county of practice are not due solely to specialization. For all three groups of specialists there is a tendency for physicians to practice in counties similar to the ones in which they grew up. Therefore, one would conclude that the selective recruitment of medical students from lower income and urban communities, which the Comprehensive Health Manpower Act encourages, would have a positive effect on the maldistribution of physicians.

At the same time, the influence of such a program in itself would be very small. This is because the effect is most pronounced among physicians who are generalists (see p. 116). And as noted previously, only 13.4 percent of the 1960 class were in general and family practice in 1972 (see p. 101). Therefore, persons most apt to be affected by a change in recruitment policy constitute only a small proportion of all physicians. In addition, the proportion of classes for later years may be even smaller. Consequently, selecting more medical school students from poorer communities would not in itself greatly influence the way physicians are now distributed in American society.

In summary, both community of origin and specialization are related to community of practice and the effect of each is independent of the effects of the other. Consequently, results support medical schools training more generalists as well as recruiting more students from low-income communities. At the same time, the influence of either program alone would be constrained by factors that are the focus of attention by the other. The effects of producing more generalists would be limited by the fact that such a small proportion of physicians originate from settings where the supply of physician manpower is low; and the effects of recruiting students from these settings would be limited by the fact that such a small proportion of medical school graduates choose careers in general medicine. A more fruitful policy would be one that combines greater emphasis on training generalists with a selective recruitment program. This becomes especially clear when the interaction effects of origin and specialization on subsequent practice setting are considered.

Interaction of Origin and Specialization

We observed earlier that if the effects of a variable, X, on Y are the same across the entire range of variable Z, the effects of variable X are additive with respect to Z. As applied to the relationship between specialization and income of county of practice (Table 12-1), the effects of specialization would be additive if the relationship between specialization and income of county of practice were the same for physicians from all origins. If, however, the effects of specialization were different for physicians of different backgrounds, the effects of specialization would interact with physician background. Results in Table 12-1 show that although there is an overall net effect (as reflected in the Partial Gamma of 0.11), the effect varies widely depending on income level of physicians' county of origin. Physicians from high income counties tend to practice in high income counties regardless of their specialty, whereas the income level for county of practice for physicians from low-income counties increases sharply from generalists to limited specialists. Therefore, the effects of specialization interact with community of origin.

Interaction is also indicated from Table 8-4 and Figure 8-1, which show that the effects of income of county of origin vary depending on level of specialization, being inverse with degree of specialization. Hence, the effects of community of origin are not additive across specialties but rather interact with specialization. The interaction is different from that revealed in Table 12-1, however, since the effects of county of origin on choice of practice setting are modified by the effects of specialization rather than the reverse. In contrast to Table 12-1, where origin is treated as an antecedant variable to specialization and county of practice, in Table 8-4 and Figure 8-1 specialization is viewed as an intervening variable that influences the relationship between origin and practice. Table 12-2 shows this relationship by the percentage of physicians who practice in a county with the same income level as their county of origin (of course, in many instances the county of origin and county of practice is the same) by specialty. The stronger tendency for generalists to practice in counties similar in income to their counties of origin is clear. For all income levels, the percentage of generalists praticing in the same or similar county as their origin is higher than the other two groups, and in all but one instance the percentage is higher for general specialists than for limited specialists. Therefore, the effects of county of origin on decisions about practice locations are greatest for generalists, weakest for limited specialists.[d]

---

[d]Results for county urban level are similar. See Table C-9 of Appendix C.

Table 12-2

Percentages of Physicians by Income of County of Origin who Practice in Counties with the Same or Similar Income, by Specialization—Class of 1960

County Income	Generalists	General Specialists	Limited Specialists	All Physicians[a]
$7,000 and above	52.2	50.0	43.9	46.3
$6,000-$6,999	56.0	46.0	50.6	49.9
$5,000-$5,999	42.1	37.7	36.2	37.4
$4,000-$4,999	38.3	30.3	18.6	25.3
$3,000-$3,999	26.5	16.3	8.5	14.9
Less than $3,000	29.0	11.1	5.3	14.6

Source: AAMC Longitudinal Study and U.S. Bureau of the Census (1967).

[a]From Table 4-2.

In summary, then, results reveal that county of origin and specialization each have effects that are independent of the other as well as effects that are dependent on those of the other. The relationships may be expressed in a formal regression model as follows:

$$P = a + b_1 (O) + b_2 (S) + b_3 (OS) + e$$

where P is the income (urbanization) of community of practice, O is income (urbanization) of community of origin, S is specialization, and e is the error term. Note, however, that the interaction term involve two processes. One is the variable effect of specialization depending on the type of community physicians come from and the other is the variable effect of community of origin depending on physician's choice of medical specialization.

Implications

As noted, medical school programs based on values for the O and S terms separately would have the effect of creating more physicians for lower income and rural counties, but the effects would not be great. Greater benefit will accrue from programs that recognize the interaction effects of origin and specialization. To influence the distribution of physician manpower, special emphasis on recruiting students from low-income, rural communities should be combined with an increased emphasis on training general physicians. Therefore, schools that attempt to modify the distribution of physicians by training more general and family practitioners should also recruit more students from low-income, rural communities. Only then will a substantial proportion of the generalist graduates be apt to locate in such communities (for example, generalists from high-income counties are as probable as specialists from those counties to locate in high-income counties, where physician manpower is already high—see Table 12-2). Results also indicate still greater success if medical schools focused their training in general and family practice on students from low-income and rural areas.

To the extent that federal manpower acts are concerned with affecting the distribution of physicians, level of funding should be consistent with what is to be expected from the program. Specifically, since the effects to be expected either from large general and family practice programs or from recruiting more students from economically depressed rural settings are quite limited, funds available for such programs should be limited accordingly. Funding at substantial levels should be reserved for schools that introduce both large programs in general and family practice *and* recruit large proportions of their students from underserved areas. Additional funding might also be granted to schools who make special efforts to direct students from low-income and rural communities into general and family practice.

These conclusions are, of course, based on results for a sample of physicians from one graduating class. Study of other graduating classes might yield different results, which could raise questions about the policy implications outlined here. At the same time, the fact that some of the findings for this class are similar to findings for all physicians, as well as for studies of other samples of physicians, gives confidence in their validity; it would seem that the above policies would rest on a fairly secure empirical base. Even so, there are serious questions about their implementation.

The identification of potential physicians from low-income, rural communities would require their identification prior to medical school, and would have to begin at least as early as the first four years of college and ideally as early as the high-school years. Also, since colleges and universities are apt to be increasingly located in the wealthier more urbanized settings in the future—to achieve the kinds of external economies that most types of organizations require (e.g., in this case, access to large numbers of potential students), the probability of a student from such a setting attending a four-year college will probably continue to be higher than that of a student from a low-income, rural area. Moreover, education in wealthier and more dense, populous counties, and especially for suburban communities, is probably going to continue to be of higher quality than that in poorer less densely populated counties. Consequently, students from these areas are probably going to be better qualified to enter college and once there, better prepared to achieve the standards necessary to enter and graduate from medical school.

In addition, getting medical school recruitment committees to select students according to their community backgrounds might prove difficult. The tendency to select students on the basis of intellectual criteria and professional promise is probably too strong to overcome easily and quickly with federal funding. And the policy of encouraging students to train for general practice depending on their community background has obvious problems. In addition, the creation of more physician manpower for underserved communities by recruiting a larger proportion of students from them might have more negative than positive consequences even for the communities themselves. It was observed that higher educated persons and persons with professional and technical occupational skills are most apt to be the types of individuals who migrate from rural areas, and the same is probably true for low-income communities. And it is certainly true of migration from the congested cities to the suburbs. The potentially negative consequences for these communities of sending a larger proportion of their sons and daughters to medical school is therefore evident. The gain in physician manpower might be at the expense of a net loss of talented persons in general. It is probable that a substantial proportion of the medical school graduates from these communities who do not return to these communities might have done so if they had not become physicians, even general and family physicians. Consequently, the process of selectively recruiting from underserved communities may, on balance, lead to an overall reduction in the proportion of persons capable of performing occupations requiring technical skills. The result might be a net loss to the community in terms of talent and overall social and economic development. Therefore, from a sociological (rather than medical) perspective, it is not clear that the recruitment of a higher proportion of students from underserved communities would make these communities (not the individuals recruited) better off than they are now.

In regard to a change in medical school emphasis on specialization, there is the question of whether such a change in emphasis is feasible or even desirable. In light of the technological and knowledge base of medicine, it will be difficult to reverse the trend toward specialization. The specialization process, once started and supported by a body of specialized knowledge, complex technology, and refined technical skills, is difficult to reverse. Efforts to do so will probably not reduce very much the institutional impulsions within medicine toward even greater specialization. The technological and knowledge base which supports and encourages medical specialization runs wide and deep. Exposure of students to continued advances in knowledge and an ever increasing number of techniques for treating more disorders effectively will probably make students and graduates feel the need to gain greater knowledge in specialized areas.

In addition, it is not at all clear that a movement to general and family practice is as desirable as some seem to think. Certainly specialty care is apt to be of higher quality if provided by the appropriate specialist than if provided by a generalist. Perhaps more thought should be directed to bringing about a greater degree of coherence and coordination in the delivery of specialty care, as discussed in Chapter 11, than to training more generalists who are able to treat a wide range of illnesses.

Career Plans

Aside from these issues, the effect of medical school experience on actual career choice of students needs to be examined. The issue is difficult to investigate, but some evidence does exist. As noted in Chapter 8, 21 percent of the 1960 class planned a career in general practice during their senior year. Certainly medical school experience orients most students in the direction of specialty practice. The question, however, is whether such orientations influence actual careers and places of practice.

The relationship between career plans and actual careers is clear from Table 12-3. Physicians who plan a career in general medicine during their senior year are far more apt to be in general and family practice 12 years later than are those who plan some form of specialty career (45.0% versus 5.7%). By the same token, those planning a specialty career are far more apt to be in a limited specialty than those who plan a career in general medicine (61.3% versus 29.9%). Without question, then, career plans during medical school predict actual careers.

But from the standpoint of the distribution of practicing physicians, the significant question concerns the relationship between career plans during the senior year and types of community setting in which physicians were practicing

Table 12-3
Relationship Between Career Plan (1960) and Actual Career (1972), in Percentages–Class of 1960

	Career Plans	
Actual Career	*General Practice*	*Specialty Practice*
Limited specialization	29.9	61.3
General specialization	25.1	33.0
General Practice	45.0	5.7
N	438	1,640
	Gamma = 0.63 (x^2 = 453; 2 *df*; $p < $ .00001)	

Source: AAMC Longitudinal Study

12 years later. While career plans do appear to be important in these decisions, their influence may not be as great as results in Table 12-3 might suggest.

First, note that Table 12-3 shows that whereas almost all of those planning specialty careers were in specialties in 1972 (61.3%were in limited specialties and 33.0% were in general specialties), less than half of those who planned careers in general practice were in general and family practice in 1972 (45.0%). Apparently experiences encountered subsequent to medical education reinforce the tendency to specialize to a much greater extent than they do the tendency to become general and family practitioners. This may be due in large measure to whether or not a graduate engages in postgraduate education, particularly if he enters a residency program. This will almost insure that he trains for a specialty since there are so few residency programs in general practice. But there is also evidence that the type of community in which practice is established may influence physicians' decisions to specialize. Table 12-4 gives the relationship between income of county of practice and specialization (no distinction is made between general and limited specialists) for only those who stated a preference for a career in general medicine during their senior year. The results are clear. Physicians who practice in higher income counties are far more apt to have changed their career plans and to be in specialty practices in 1972. For example, 82.0 percent of those practicing in counties with incomes below \$4,000 were in general and family practice and 18.0 percent in specialty practice, in contrast to 36.5 and 63.5 percent who were practicing in counties with incomes of \$7,000

Table 12-4

Relationship Between Specialization and Income of County of Practice for Physicians Who Planned General Practice Careers in 1960

	Income of County of Practice (1960)				
Specialty in 1972	*Below* *$4,000*	*$4,000-* *$4,999*	*$5,000-* *$5,999*	*$6,000-* *$6,999*	*$7,000* *and Above*
Specialty[a]	18.0	48.5	60.2	62.2	63.5
Generalist	82.0	51.5	39.8	37.8	36.5
N	50	66	113	127	63

Gamma = 0.30 (x^2 = 34; 4 df; $p < .0001$)

Sources: AAMC Longitudinal Study and U.S. Bureau of the Census (1967).

[a]Includes limited and general specialties.

and above.[e] There is no way to know which came first—the change in career
plan or selection of a county of practice. It is possible that a change in career
plan influenced choice of county rather than the reverse. It is probable, however,
that for a substantial proportion choice of practice setting preceded the change
in career.

Finally, the possible influence of career plans versus actual careers in determining practice setting needs to be considered. In Chapter 8 the relationship
between community of origin and community of practice was examined separately for the three specialty groups, thus "controlling" or minimizing the effects of
specialization. As noted, results showed that the strength of the origin-practice
relationship is inversely related to specialization, being strongest for general and
family practitioners. This is due to generalists from low-income, rural communities being more inclined to practice in similar communities than are specialists
from such communities, and general specialists are more apt to do so than limited
specialists from these communities. These relationships were presented in Table
8-4. Now if career attitudes during the senior year also have an influence, corresponding differences should exist. That is, the relationship between community
of origin and community of practice should be stronger for those who plan
general practice careers than for those who aspire to more specialized careers.
This in fact is the case. The correlation and regression coefficients (r and b) are
0.47 and 0.432 respectively for those with general practice career plans (GPCP)
but only 0.36 and 0.317 for those who plan specialty careers (SCP) (see Table
12-5, bottom row). Table 12-5 presents the correlation coefficient, regression
coefficient and intercept for the relationship between income for county of
origin and income for county of practice separately for those who intended a
career in general practice (GPCP) and those who intended a career in more
specialized practice (SCP). This table is similar to the upper part of Table 8-4
except that results for each of the three specialty groups are presented for two
separate groups depending on their career intentions during the senior year.

Comparison of r's, b's, and a's for physicians in the same specialty group
who had different career plans may be made across rows (e.g., the r for physicians in limited specialties in 1972 who planned careers in general practice
in 1960 is 0.38 in comparison to an r of 0.30 for limited specialists who
planned specialty careers). Such comparisons indicate the effect of place of
origin on place of practice for physicians who had different career plans with
actual level of specialization controlled. Although there are differences between
the coefficients, the only meaningful pattern is in the a coefficient, which reveals that for each specialty group, those who expressed the intention to specialize tend to come from somewhat wealthier counties than those who expressed
an intention to enter general practice.

---

[e]Results are similar for urbanization. See Table C-10 of Appendix C.

Table 12-5

Correlation Coefficient (r), Regression Coefficient (b), and Intercept (a) for the Relationship Between Income for County of Origin and Income of County for Practice (with County of Origin as Dependent Variable), by Career Plans and Specialty

	r		b		a		N	
	GPCP[a]	SCP[b]	GPCP	SCP	GPCP	SCP	SPCP	SCP
Limited specialists	0.38	0.30	0.294	0.261	$4,448	$4,756	117	923
General specialists	0.42	0.37	0.366	0.342	$3,914	$4,247	99	497
Generalists	0.53	0.62	0.504	0.558	$2,675	$2,960	186	84
Totals	0.47	0.36	0.432	0.317	$3,336	$4,369	402	1,504

Source: AAMC Longitudinal Study and U.S. Bureau of the Census (1967).

[a]GPCP = General Practice Career Plans.

[b]SCP = Specialty Career Plan.

Comparison of coefficients within columns indicate the effect of place of origin on place of practice for different specialty groups with career plans controlled. Regardless of career plans, the r's and b's are highest for generalists and lowest for limited specialists; the pattern of difference is virtually the same for those who had general practice career plans (GPCP) as for those who had specialty career plans (SCP). Moreover, the pattern for each of the two groups is almost identical to that for both groups combined in Table 8-4. Therefore, controlling for career plan has no apparent influence on the effect actual specialization exerts on the relationship between income of origin and income of practice. This means, in effect, that medical school efforts to instill generalist career orientations among their students may have little if any effect unless those plans are actually implemented. And the implementation of such plans is, to a substantial degree, beyond the control of medical schools.

Of course, since career plans and actual plans are themselves rather highly correlated (see Table 12-3), control for actual career also controls to some extent for career plan. Thus it might be argued that control for both of these variables should lead to different results than when only one is controlled. However, the results in Table 12-5 where both are controlled are only slightly different from those when only actual specialization is controlled (Table 8-4). And the difference between results when only career plan is controlled (totals row of Table 12-5) and when both are controlled (internal cells) is considerable.

It would seem, then, that in themselves, career plans, at least as developed by the end of the senior year, do not substantially affect the relationship between physician county of origin and county of practice; type of career plan, in itself, does not influence the tendency of physicians to practice in communities similar to those in which they were reared. This obviously raises questions as to how much influence undergraduate medical education may have on the distribution of physicians in the United States. This is not to say, of course, that instilling general practice career orientations among medical students would have no effect. It probably does since it contributes to level of specialization even when community of origin is controlled. However, to the extent that it does not result in actual career choice, career plan seems to have little effect on where a physician locates his practice. Moreover, specialization is the product of things other than just medical education and career plans that are based on it. The argument, therefore, is that (1) the success of medical schools in developing general rather than speciality orientations is constrained by student experience prior to medical education, and (2) the effects of those orientations, once adopted, on where a physician locates his practice is constrained both by the types of community experiences he encountered prior to medical education and the types of community experiences he has once his education has been completed. Medical schools have little control over such external experiences.

Conclusion

It is axiomatic that before one becomes a physician one must receive a medical education. Yet this experience is not the sole determinant of the maldistribution of physicians. The distribution of physicians is also a product of more general societal processes such as were outlined in previous chapters. The choice of community of practice is in large part determined by the social, economic, and demographic differences between communities that make communities more or less attractive to physicians and by difference in community of origin. Medical schools can do little to modify these forces. However, the training of more general and family practitioners in combination with a program that recruits a higher proportion of students from underserved areas would probably lead to a more even distribution than now exists. Whether such programs represent viable alternatives for medical schools is an open question, however. It is not clear that the trend toward specialization can or even should be reversed and the same is true for changing medical-school policy of recruiting students on the basis of academic and professional criteria. This aside, the effects of such programs will be constrained by the broader context of forces that have their locus in social and economic differences between communities, and over which medical schools have little if any control.

13

Increasing the Supply of Manpower and Equalizing Economic Demand

In contrast to changing the types of physicians recruited and produced, other programs are concerned with increasing the supply of manpower. The approach is examined in this chapter. Programs that would make the economic demand for medical care more equal are also examined.

Increasing the Overall Supply of Physicians

From one point of view the uneven distribution of physicians in communities in the United States is one of numbers: There are fewer in some communities than in others. This is not to say that all communities should have the same physician-to-population ratio or that all communities should have the same identical range of services; this obviously would entail considerable waste—both of physician manpower and of economic resources. Probably no one recommends this. Still, there are communities where shortages of physicians are acute and very few (if any) communities where most community members believe the community has too many physicians. Consequently, some believe that a change in the distribution of physicians must come about by increasing the supply of physicians.

Increasing the overall supply of physicians and, hence, an increase in the number of medical students—either by expanding current medical schools or establishing new ones[a]—would appear to be a rather straightforward solution to the maldistribution problem. This is particularly the case if it is assumed that efforts of the medical profession to restrict the supply of physicians is one of the major (if not the major) factors that has caused the maldistribution problem. Advocates of this approach apparently assume that if the number of physicians increase, physicians will be gradually pushed out into rural and economically deprived areas or pushed into the inner cities to practice. The assumption is valid—at some point. Beyond some point increases in the number of physicians in high manpower environments will lead to the movement of physicians out of

---

[a]The Carnegie Commission presented a plan for medical schools to produce 50 more physicians by 1980 over 1970. *Carnegie Commission on Higher Education, Higher Education and the Nation's Health: Policies for Medical and Dental Education*, New York: McGraw-Hill, 1970. A total of nineteen new medical schools were established between 1965 and 1972 and the size of the entering class for all medical schools increased 46 percent (National Academy of Sciences 1974, p. 57).

175

such areas or of physicians establishing their initial practices in areas where physicians are in short supply.

The basic question is economic: Can the United States afford to educate enough physicians so that a substantial number are unable to make a living (or a very good one) by practicing in areas where physicians are in ample supply, so that they will locate elsewhere? If the answer to this question is positive, then the solution to the distributional problem could be solved by increasing the supply of physicians. The question is difficult to answer, for two reasons.

First, the number of additional physicians required before physicians would be forced into areas where shortages exist is hard to estimate. It is probable that the required number would be considerable. Second, since the number of additional graduates needed to provide sufficient manpower in currently underserved areas is not known, it is hard to estimate what the cost would be. Current figures on the cost of medical education do not warrant encouragement. The report of a study of the *Costs of Education in the Health Professions* by the National Academy of Sciences (1974) reveals a range of $6,900 to $18,650 in the annual cost per student among the schools studied (1974, p. 62). Income from tuition and fees provide a very small proportion of total medical school income from all sources (education, patient care, research)—from 2 percent to 4 percent for public schools and from 3 percent to 11 percent for private schools (the average for private schools is 5.6%) (National Academy of Sciences 1974, pp. 94-95). Consequently, the expense of educating more medical students would have to be borne mostly by the taxpayer and private contributors. An exact interpretation of such figures is difficult because the figures include expenditures for research, service (patient care), and administration, as well as teaching costs. At the same time, these nonteaching expenditures are essential to medical education. Whether the proportion of such expenditures can or should be reduced is another matter. But even if they were reduced, their total elimination would not be desirable, or even feasible. Also, the cost of training more medical students is difficult to estimate because such costs will undoubtedly vary depending on whether enrollments in existing medical schools increase or whether new medical schools are established. (Existing schools do not incur the expense of start-up costs and they can realize the economies of scale associated with increased size of operation.) But in any case, most will agree that the cost of medical education is expensive; the total expenditure would increase with an increase in the number of students. Such costs would, at some point, restrain the expansion of existing medical schools and the establishment of new ones.

On balance, an increase in medical school graduates would not be expected to lead to greater equity in the distribution of physicians. In the first place, some increase will be required just to keep up with population growth; before the physician-to-population ratio increases, the number of physician graduates must increase faster than the population grows. In addition, a larger supply of physicians will very likely continue to be patterned on the same community characteristics that is now the case, so that the relative difference between communities will not likely be modified by an increase in the overall physician-to-population ratios. There are several reasons for this.

A community's supply of physicians is a component of the professional service sector, and this is interrelated with economic and demographic factors, including suburbanization. Changes in the distribution of physicians as a result of a larger overall supply will be constrained by the amount of change in these factors. Even if an increase in the number of physicians does reduce the income of many physicians in areas currently characterized by high physician-population ratios, there are other factors to keep physicians in these communities and to attract others to them. Also, specialists are more apt than generalists to concentrate in more populous affluent communities. Although efforts are being made to create a viable speciality of family medicine, which some hope will largely replace the function of general practitioner, the extent to which programs in family medicine will proliferate in medical schools, and for how long, are unanswered questions. Moreover, there is no guarantee that *specialists* in family medicine will choose to practice in communities now characterized by low physician-to-population ratios. Futhermore, results in Chapter 9 showed that the distribution of general and family practitioners is substantially influenced by the suburbanization process, and thus suggest that the suburbs will gain in their supply of these physicians with inner cities and possibly low-income rural communities losing ground.

If there develops an excessive supply of physicians in areas currently characterized by high physician manpower, one can always argue that physicians in these communities, even those who are limited specialists, may seek their livelihood in underserved areas. It is probable, however, that it will take more than a reduction in income to move large numbers of physicians from advantaged to disadvantaged communities. It is hard to believe that many of the limited specialists will ever be forced or pushed out into rural communities where their special skills would find little use.[b] Moreover, the economic costs of producing an excessive supply of physicians—enough to effect the distribution of physicians—would be extremely high, and they are probably prohibitive. Indeed, it may be very expensive just to keep the absolute physician manpower level in many low ratio communities from dropping lower than is now the case.

It will be enlightening to review some findings reported in Chapter 3 (p. 52). In spite of an almost constant physician-to-population ratio for the entire nation from 1923 to 1938, Joseph W. Mountin and associates report

---

[b]Also, primary-care physicians may be reluctant to practice in the inner city with the congestion, impersonality, and anonymity that characterize life there. Such an atmosphere is not conducive to the development of interpersonal relationships between patient and physician that many believe are essential in patient relationships with primary-care providers, especially general and family practitioners.

that considerable change occurred among counties, and that the change was systematically associated with county wealth (Mountin, Pennell, and Nicolay 1942c, p. 1947). Also, the number of counties without at least one practicing physician increased from 1950 to 1971: 64 in 1950; 74 in 1959; 98 in 1963; 126 in 1967; and 133 in 1971. This occurred in spite of an apparent overall *in*crease in the national physician manpower ratio: In 1950, according to the U.S. Census, there were 127 employed physicians (this includes federal physicians except those in the armed forces) per 100,000 United States resident population (Pennell and Altenderfer 1954, p. 7); in 1971, according to the results of the American Medical Association annual questionnaire, there were 143 active nonfederal and federal physicians (excluding those in the armed forces) per 100,000 population (Roback 1972, pp. 3, 4, 7). Nevertheless, the supply of physicians in many communities was lower in 1971 than in 1950.

What these results reveal is that the distribution of physicians is not necessarily a function of total numbers (or overall physician-to-population ratio). For two periods, one in which the overall ratio was constant and one in which there was an apparent substantial increase, a serious manpower problem existed in more communities at the end of the period than at the beginning. This does not mean that increases in physician manpower will inevitably lead to more serious distributional problems, of course; history does not always repeat itself. At the same time, history cautions against optimism that an increased supply will either reduce the severity of the distributional problem (which is a matter of relative differences between communities) or even that it will lead to an increase in the absolute manpower situation in communities where the most severe manpower problems currently exist.

Increases in the supply of medical manpower as a solution to the maldistribution of physicians are not limited to programs for increasing the supply of physicians. Programs for training more allied health personnel have also been recommended, especially the training of physician's assistants.

Physician's Assistants

A number of educational and training programs are currently underway to train persons to perform many of the duties now performed by physicans. These are called by a variety of names, such as Medex programs, which are designed to provide additional training for the returning military medic; Primex programs, which upgrade the skills of the registered nurse so she/ he can function as a nurse clinician; and others, which are simply called physician's assistants programs. All have in common the belief that many of the duties of physicians are routine and do not require the in-depth and range of medical knowledge that physicians possess. It is believed, therefore, that physician's assistants can be trained to perform many of the activities physicians now perform. Although the original conception of physician's assistant seemed to be that this person would be trained primarily to assist general practitioners, more specialized programs have developed, such as orthopedic assistant, urologic physician's assistant, and pediatric nurse practitioners. The underlying conception in all programs, however, is that with the support of physician's assistants, physicians will be able to extend their reach and see many more patients than they now have the capacity to see (Sadler, Sadler, and Bliss 1972). The development of physician's assistants has been hailed as "in many respects . . . the most exciting health manpower innovation in several decades." It "is exciting because it holds great promise for improving and distributing health care" (Sadler, Sadler, and Bliss 1972, p. 9). Rashi Fein also thinks the use of paramedics has great promise for providing health in areas of physician shortage (1967, pp. 90-129; see also Marshall et al. 1971, p. 1563).

Many questions surround the development of physician's assistant programs. They include problems of licensure and certification in various states and how these are to be uniform among the states; problems of proper supervision; questions as to the quality of health care such persons are capable of delivering; and what will happen to the many persons (many of whom are nurses) who are actually now operating as (uncertified) physician's assistants, especially as the newly trained physician's assistants become professionalized and concerned about outsiders infringing on their professional domain.

These and other questions cloud the issue of this new occupation. The concern here, however, is with another question; namely, what is the probability that physician's assistants will establish and maintain their practice in the kinds of communities that are now characterized by low physician ratios? Results in Chapter 3 revealed that other professionally trained persons nationwide, as well as registered nurses in one state, tend to concentrate in counties that are high in socioeconomic characteristics. One may well ask if professional persons, such as nurse clinicians, are going to locate in low supply areas with any greater frequency once they have received more professional training. It is almost (if not quite) like saying that if a general practitioner receives more training in order to become a specialist, he will be more inclined to locate in areas now characterized by low physician manpower. The same question may be raised of the former corpman (Medex). What is he going to find in such communities that other professional and semiprofessional persons, in and out of the medical field, have been unable to find? The question raised by Clifford L. Carlson and Gary T. Athelstan is to the point: "How will overlaying this distorted pattern of [physician manpower] distribution with a parallel distribution of physician's assistants produce meaningful advantages for medically deprived persons and areas?" (Carlson and Athelstan 1970, p. 1855).

In this connection, the results of a study of general hospitals are informative. In a survey of 105 general hospitals (all members of the American Hospital Association) in the Tennessee Mid-South region, I was able in 1969 to obtain information on the number of personnel in each of several occupational categories for 91 of these hospitals.[c] Occupational categories include the number of registered nurses, practical nurses and nurse technicians, and aides-orderlies, expressed as the number per 100 beds. A comparison of the correlation coefficients and regression slopes for median family income (1959) for the county in which the hospital is located is presented in Figure 13-1. The results are clear: The effect of community income on health manpower varies directly with the professional development and technical expertise of the occupation. But even the semiskilled practical nurses and nurse technicians tend to be concentrated in the more affluent counties, though slightly less so than registered nurses. Is it not implausible to assume that physician's assistants will be able to find employment in high income areas as easily as practical nurses? Indeed, if the concept of physician's assistant is viable and such persons are able to provide needed services which enable physicians to see more patients or at least be relieved of some pressure from patient demands, what is there to prevent physicians in richer environments, where the physician ratios are high but where many persons still have limited access to medical care, from utilizing physician's assistants? Such communities would probably be more attractive to physician's assistants than those communities where services are currently in shortest supply.

In addition, to the extent that physician's assistants become a major element in American medicine, it is not unlikely that in their development they will follow the course of physician specialization; physician's assistants will be trained to assist particular specialists among physicians. Carlson and Athelstan observe that: "Much current activity is concentrated on creating assistants who are 'custom designed' to serve a single specialty" and note that 66 programs in existence or under development as of December 1970 were training pediatric nurse practitioners (Carlson and Athelstan 1970, p. 1855). To the extent that the physician's assistant is trained to be an assistant, he is limited in his locational patterns to the locational patterns of physicians. And since specialists tend to locate in the more affluent populous areas, this will be a significant factor in the locational pattern of physician's assistants.

This is not a recommendation against physician's assistants programs. The distribution of manpower is only one criterion against which such programs should be assessed—though I suspect it is too frequently considered the primary consideration. There are other potential benefits. These include purely economic and occupational ones, in which employment opportunities would be

---

[c]For a description of the survey, see Bruce H. Mayhew and William A. Rushing (1973). The Tennessee Mid-South region encompasses those counties identified with the Tennessee Mid-South Regional Medical Program. The region includes 74 counties in Middle and East Tennessee (counties lying East of the West transection of the Tennessee River in Tennessee) and 13 counties in Southwest Kentucky.

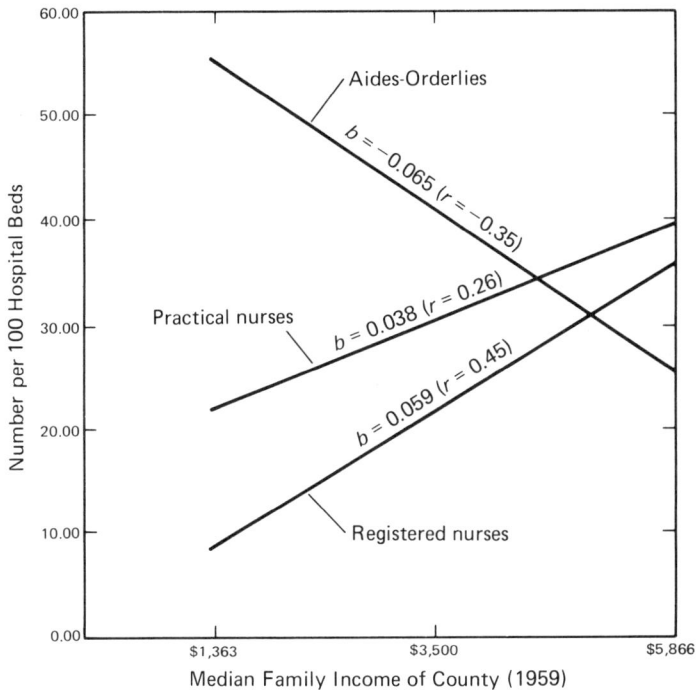

Figure 13-1. Regression of Three Nursing Ratios on County Median Family Income for Hospitals in the Tennessee Mid-South Region

opened and career ladders extended for returning military corpsmen, registered nurses, and other health-care personnel whose career opportunities are truncated by a low ceiling on upward mobility within their respective occupations. My less than enthusiastic endorsement of physician's assistants is in terms of the impact, or lack of impact, that I expect them to have on the distribution of health-care manpower.

Conclusion

Efforts to reduce the magnitude of the maldistribution problem through an increase in numbers fail to consider that the current supply of physicians in some of the higher income, more urban communities do not meet the demand for medical care in as optimum a manner as many community members desire. Complaints of excessive queuing, impersonal treatment, and expensive care in comparatively rich communities are not at all unusual; the major benefit of an increased supply of physicians and allied health personnel may be less waiting, less impersonal treatment, better care and lower costs for citizens of *advantaged* communities. When we also consider that the supply of medical care creates to some degree its own demand (Ginzburg and Ostow 1969), an increase in the overall supply of medical manpower may lead in fact to an increased demand in communities where medical manpower is already high. Also, increases in the overall supply do not influence the community *differences* in demand, which are associated with "demand characteristics" of communities.

Toward Equalizing Demand: Universal Health Insurance

If the ability to purchase medical care were made more equal through some form of universal health insurance, the differences between communities in the sheer economic demand for medical care would be reduced. Many believe that some form of health insurance will be available in the near future to all citizens of the United States, provided either by private insurance carriers or government sponsorship. Government insurance programs for health are controversial, and I won't discuss the pros and cons of such programs here. Concern is only with the probable consequence universal health insurance will have for the distribution of physicians in communities throughout the United States.

At first thought one would expect that it would make for a more even distribution of physicians. This assumes that a major factor in the maldistribution of physicians is economic motivation; therefore, if the demand for medical care in poor environments is raised through third-party payers, physicians would be more apt to locate their practice in such environments. The argument is faulty in several respects.

In the first place, the assumption that the distribution of physicians is determined by a rather simplistic monetary motive is to be questioned. As argued earlier, it is probable that the maldistribution of physicians is more a function of physicians' search for occupational opportunity than of economic motivation per se. If this is so, then a change in the distribution of economic demand for medical care without corresponding changes in community settings that influence physicians' opportunity to pursue the kind of practice most have been trained to provide will not go very far toward modifying the existing community inequities in physician manpower.

In addition, surveys of physicians from disadvantaged areas suggest that cultural and social differences between advantaged and disadvantaged communities are factors in their choosing the latter over the former (cf. Bible 1970; Crawford and McCormack 1971). Although these factors may be less important than those associated with occupational opportunity (see pp. 109), to the extent that they *are* involved, greater equalization of the demand for medical care through universal health insurance will certainly do little to change them. An insurance program will have virtually no influence on the cultural opportunities, recreational and educational facilities, and quality of life that communities have to offer.

Other causal factors are differences between communities in socialization institutions that lead to community differences in the production rates of physicians. This along with the apparent desire to locate in a setting similar in social and economic characteristics to the one in which one was reared leads to a greater supply of physicians in communities that produce more physicians. This is a function of differences in community institutions, and policies that reduce community differences in the economic demand for medical care do not effect these differences.

But the argument that universal health insurance will help to redress the maldistribution of physicians may be defective in a more basic respect. It ignores that such a program will increase the demand for medical care in almost all communities, not just the underserved communities. First, there are probably many persons in populous, affluent communities who are financially able to purchase medical care but who do not purchase it as frequently as they would if they had insurance coverage; with such coverage, their purchases will increase.[d] Second, even in most high income areas there is a significant proportion of the population for whom financial barriers to the purchase of medical care are quite serious. Even in most wealthy areas there are places (slums, ghettos) in which the level of living is quite low, and where the inhabitants receive little medical attention. Results in Chapter 6 show that within urban areas physicians concentrate in the suburban communities. The results of others have also shown that the distribution of physicians in various sections of cities is correlated with the income characteristics of those sections, with physician ratios being higher in higher income areas (Star 1971; Terris and Monk 1956, pp. 588-89). When physicians have the choice of locating their practice in poor sections of urban areas and residing in more attractive sections (e.g., the suburbs) or locating their practice *and* residence in low-income, rural communities, it is reasonable to expect that they will choose the former. Most physicians would probably rather treat middle-class patients than lower class patients; but given little difference between the class mix of patients, physicians will tend to locate in settings that will afford them professional contact with physician colleagues and social contact, for themselves as well as their families, with persons from the stream of middle-class

---

[d]There is less evidence concerning the effect of health insurance on the demand for nonhospital services than for hospital services. However, one study does report a major increase in physician contacts in the Baltimore area as a result of medicaid (Bice 1971), and in an unpublished study of two rural communities in Southern Appalachia the author and David L. Miles find that the influence of insurance on the purchase of physician services is not limited to low income families by any means. (See Rushing and Miles 1975.)

society. It is not likely, therefore, that universal health insurance will provide sufficient economic or noneconomic incentives for physicians to locate in the generally economically declining rural communities now characterized by low physician ratios. It may increase the demand for physician services to such an extent that many additional physicians will be supported in those environments now characterized by high physician ratios, with the inner cities finding some relief as a result.

In addition, the increased demand in low-income rural areas may actually reduce the supply of physicians in these areas. There is evidence that physicians in low manpower areas already see more patients and work longer hours than their counterparts in higher manpower areas (cf. Bible 1970; Crawford and McCormack 1971; Fein 1967; Parker and Tuxhill 1967; Rimlinger and Steele 1963). Also, one study reports that the primary reason physicians from large communities give for not locating in rural communities is the work load in the latter (Parker and Tuxhill 1967). Further, the percentage appears to have increased over time, or at least it increases depending on year of medical school graduation: from 26.2 percent and 21.8 percent for 1919-29 and 1930-39 graduates to 42.6 percent for physicians who graduated during the 1956-64 period (Parker and Tuxhill 1967). With an increase in demand in low manpower areas, the problem is apt to grow worse. Already there are reports, and the author knows of several cases, in which medicare and medicaid have resulted in demands that physicians from rural, low-income communities have felt unable to absorb. In consequence, some physicians have moved to areas where the manpower problem is less acute and the pressure of patient demand is not as great. How general this is no one can say; but since these programs have led to an increase in demand in rich, as well as poor, environments, there is reason to expect that it has occurred in many instances and, with the introduction of universal insurance coverage, that it will occur in many more instances in the future.

Therefore, although universal health insurance may alleviate problems of inequity at the individual level (since differences in the ability to purchase medical care are reduced) and possibly for some places in large cities, it is not likely to reduce inequities between geographic areas of different income and urbanization levels. In terms of these differences, the distributional problem may actually get worse. This is so because physicians will have even less incentive to live in these less attractive communities. Although insurance coverage may assure physicians a thriving practice even in economically deprived communities, physicians will have still greater incentive to locate in more attractive communities because of the unmet economic demand there. Thus, efforts to solve the distributional problem at the individual level may make the problem at the community level worse.

Conclusion

Increases in the supply of physician manpower or the reduction of inequities in the demand for health care are not apt to have a major positive effect on the maldistribution of physicians. Increases in supply fail to change differences between communities in general social and economic characteristics which are so important in the distribution of physician manpower. Consequently, increases in supply will not likely modify the current relationships between community characteristics and physician manpower. Moreover, since the supply of physician manpower may create its own demand, an increase in the supply may increase the demand for medical care in areas where physician manpower is considered to be in ample supply. The effect of equalizing demand is limited in that it does nothing about causes of the maldistribution that are apparently unrelated to the economic motivation of physicians. These include institutional differences in communities that lead to differential productivity rates, physician preference to practice in setting resembling the community in which one was reared, and the concern for social and cultural opportunities for oneself and one's family. In addition, however, there are probably many persons in high-income, urban communities who may not purchase medical care as much as they would if the out-of-pocket costs were less than they are now. Insurance coverage would make such persons more disposed to obtain care and hence allow for the economic support of an even larger supply of physicians in communities where the supply is already comparatively high.

14 Changing the Location of Training Institutions

Some believe that changes in the location of places where physicians are educated and trained would influence where they subsequently practice. Specifically, it is argued that if more training institutions were located in communities where the supply of physicians is in short supply, the supply of physicians in those communities would increase. In examining this position, the location of medical schools and residency programs will be considered separately.

Location of Medical Schools

The idea of locating medical schools in underserved areas may be a central issue when a state decides to increase the number of medical school graduates. The question is debated as to whether the best policy is to build a new medical school in an area of low physician manpower or to expand an existing school. The matter may be largely political and relate more to which areas and institutions in the state are to get additional state funds and facilities than to whether the additional facilities will contribute to meeting the medical needs of the state. However, advocates for locating medical schools in underserved areas sometimes rationalize their position in terms of the assumption that where a physician goes to medical school is a major factor in where he chooses to practice. Evidence from research studies that show that the location of a physician's practice is often the same as the location of his training (Breisch 1970; Martin, et al. 1968; and Weiskotten, et al. 1960) sometimes is cited as support for the assumption, and hence for the location of medical schools in underserved areas. In light of the evidence, the approach would appear to be a rather straightforward approach to the maldistribution problem. The evidence needs to be examined.

Contrary to popular belief, the number of medical students enrolled in a state bears very little relationship to the number of practicing physicians in a state. The product-moment correlation between the 1967 state physician ratio and the average annual number of medical school enrollees in the state per million state population for the years 1958-68 is only 0.20 for the 48 contiguous states and the District of Columbia.[a] Such results are consistent with the

---

[a]Source of data: C.N. Theodore, G.E. Sutter, and J.N. Haug (1968) and American Medical Association (1959-1967a, 1968). A 10-year average is obtained to eliminate a rate

conclusions of Rashi Fein and Gerald I. Weber, who state that "to a large extent, the success of a state in attracting physicians is independent of the number of physicians trained in its schools . . . . The ability of states to attract new physicians is only marginally improved by increases in the number of physicians graduated from medical schools in the state" (Fein and Weber 1971, pp. 159, 162).

Tennessee exemplifies the problem. For the 10-year period, 1958-68, the annual average number of enrollees in Tennessee schools was 7.91 per 100,000 population, which gave the state a rank of fourth among all states.[b] In contrast there were a total of 1,737 new physicians in Tennessee for 1955-67, for an annual average ratio of 4.37 per 100,000 and a rank of 29 among states.[c] Statistics from two years illustrate the situation. In 1967, 240 students graduated from Tennessee medical schools but only 88 new physicians were granted licenses, for a ratio of 2.72 graduates per new Tennessee physician; in 1968 the ratio was 1.89 (American Medical Association 1968, p. 1098, and *Medical Economics* 1969, pp. 100-101). In both years only one state had a higher ratio (Georgia in 1968 and Illinois in 1968).

Within states, pressure may develop to locate a medical school in an area where the physician manpower is in low supply. The rationale for these proposals seems to be that the additional medical school graduates will tend to practice in areas of the state where they are most needed. But just as there is no guarantee that graduates of a state school will remain in the state, there is no guarantee that a graduate of a school in a subregion of the state will establish his practice in that subregion. Again, Tennessee illustrates the problem. Cheatham County, which is adjacent to Davidson County where there are two medical schools (Meharry and Vanderbilt) and a high physician-to-population ratio (207 in patient care per 100,000 population in 1971),[d] reports only one physician for a population of over 13,000 (*Nashville Tennessean* 1973, p. 13); and several other counties near Davidson County have reported serious problems in attracting and keeping physicians. Similarly, Fayette County, which is adjacent to Shelby County, where the largest medical school enrollment in the Southeast (University of Tennessee) is located, has only one physician per 3,669 population (Office of Comprehensive Health Planning, Tennessee, 1970, p. 30). The two

---

for a state that is usually high or low for any one year. For example, some states with medical schools in 1968 did not have them in 1959. Figures only for 1968 would fail to show that some figures may be unusual in light of the history of various states. The Spearman rank correlation (rho) is 0.39.

[b]Source of data: C.N. Theodore, G.E. Sutter, and J.N. Haug (1968); U.S. Bureau of the Census (1964).

[c]Source of data: Theodore, Sutter, and Haug (1968, pp. 313-454); U.S. Bureau of the Census (1964).

[d]G.A. Roback (1972), pp. 286-87. The ratio is slightly inflated because population figures are for 1970 and the number of physicians is for 1971.

subregions of the state with the lowest ratios, the Upper Cumberland and South Central, are in Middle Tennessee and all counties in these two areas are located no more than one and one-half to two hours drive from Nashville, the seat of two of the three state medical schools. In the 21-county Western area, where the University of Tennessee Medical College is located, only two counties have more than 1 physician per 1,000 population and 15 have less than 1 per 2,000. Clearly, the existence of a medical school in a subregion of the state does not guarantee that all counties in the subregion will have available to them the number of physicians that the citizens in those counties may consider desirable.

This is not surprising. It is the nature of communities—their population base, economic development, and access to hospital facilities—as well as the physician's community background and level of specialization that influence where a physician establishes and continues his practice. Moreover, there are too many other factors associated with medical education—such as place of internship and residency—to conclude that the region within a state where one graduates from medical school has a major influence on the specific place he chooses to practice.

It is true, of course, that communities with medical schools also have high physician-to-population ratios. One explanation sometimes given for this is that medical schools, with the educational and other personnel and facilities, provide the professional association and support that physicians desire. (Another explanation, of course, is that in many statistics physicians on the medical school staff are included in the count.) There may be some truth to the idea that medical schools lead physicians to establish their practice in the area, but the major factor attracting both medical schools and practicing physicians is, I suspect, the social and economic character of the surrounding area. Medical schools are not located in isolated rural areas for much the same reasons that most practicing physicians are not located there. In the academic year 1971-72 there were 94 medical schools in the United States.[e] Examination shows that virtually all are affiliated with a metropolitan area. Thus, medical schools tend to be located in communities with populations large and dense enough to provide sufficient clinical material on which medical education can thrive. Indeed, in their study of academic health centers in the United States, Carter, et al., note that although "a number of factors influence the supply of teaching patients, the most straight-forward [is] population density of the area where the medical center is located" (1974:17).[f] (Carter et al. 1974, p. 19.) They find that schools located in areas where the supply of patients is restricted are more apt to

---

[e]American Medical Association (1972).

[f]The population constraint is less severe in schools in which the thrust is "almost solely in the secondary and tertiary care setting of a large referral hospital," but "the more a medical school emphasizes training in primary care and ambulatory care, the more binding will be the population constraint" (Carter et al. 1974, p. 19).

experience financial difficulties than schools located in areas where the supply is not restricted (Carter et al. 1974, pp. 66-68).[g] One may well question the wisdom of locating medical schools in areas where the physician manpower is in short supply—and where population size and density will not provide a large number and wide variety of teaching patients.[h]

Location of Residency Programs

One of the most frequently mentioned methods for redistributing physicians focuses on residency programs. The idea appears to have had its origin in the early sixties and to be based on the findings of the Weiskotten study concerning the relative importance of various factors in determining the states where 1950 medical school graduates were practicing in 1959 (Weiskotten et al. 1960). Herman G. Weiskotten et al. found that 59.3 percent were practicing in their home state where they attended medical school; 48.8 percent were practicing in the state where internship requirements were fulfilled; and 63.1 percent had located in the state of residency training. On this basis many persons have considered location of residency training to be the most significant factor in determining state of practice.

The evidence is not overly compelling, however. The difference between nativity and residency is quite small. Also, while place of residency does appear to be more important than state of medical school, the effect of residency may not be great in light of the observation that the number of state medical school students per capita and the state physician ratio are not closely related.[i] In

---

[g]Because of the measurement used for supply of patients (student-population ratio), the finding could be due to the fact that schools experiencing financial difficulties are located in areas where there are many medical schools (Carter et al. 1974, pp. 66-68).

[h]The general problem bears directly on the plan of the federal government to finance several new medical schools in conjunction with affiliated Veterans Administration hospitals. Two matters are involved. One relates to the type of communities in which the chosen hospitals are located. The success of the school will no doubt depend on the kinds of economic, demographic and social factors that have been emphasized in this book. In addition, the wisdom of using Veterans Administration hospitals for training physicians, especially primary care physicians, is most questionable. The range of illnesses necessary for training many types of physicians is simply not represented in the patient population. The population is almost 100 percent male. In addition, the potential population served (29 million veterans) is aging. Consequently, unless the United States enters another war in the near future, veterans hospitals will be increasingly concerned with domiciliary and long-term chronic care of males. Although such a population may provide good training grounds for persons specializing in geriatrics, it does not present good opportunities for training most primary-care and specialty physicians.

[i]Moreover, it is important to know what proportion of physicians were natives of the state where they did their residency and whether they attended medical school there (Yett and Sloan 1971).

addition, recommendations based on the data of the Weiskotten study (or similar data) assume that increases in the internship-resident positions lead to or cause increases in the physician ratio. It is just as plausible to argue that medical school graduates choose to do their residency in the state where they subsequently plan to practice. Indeed, Fein and Weber state: "Because of licensing factors and the need to develop contacts and a reputation, it would be logical for physicians to take their residency training in the state in which they plan to practice . . . " (Fein and Weber 1971, p. 157).

Evidence does indicate that interns-residents and physicians tend to be concentrated in the same communities. A common interpretation is that physicians tend to locate their practice in areas in which they completed their medical education (Reskin and Campbell 1974, p. 989); that is, a large supply of interns and residents in a community leads to a large supply of practicing physicians. But, as noted, the relationship may be due to individuals training in areas where they plan to practice—"the urban training site may be selected by urban-oriented students" (Cooper, Heald, and Samuels 1972, p. 940). In addition, it is at least as plausible to contend that a large supply of physicians in a community tends to lead to a large supply of interns and residents rather than the reverse. This is so because the concentration of practicing physicians is a requirement for residency and internship programs: There must be a medical faculty. Without a faculty to train interns and residents there can be no interns and residents. In Tennessee, for example, the highest physician ratios are in Davidson (Nashville) and Shelby (Memphis) counties; in 1970 these counties had approximately 87 percent of the internships in the state and 86 percent of the residencies (Tennessee Higher Education Commission 1971, p. 31). Moreover, when three other high physician ratio counties are included— Anderson (Oak Ridge), which ranks 7th, and Hamilton (Chattanooga) and Knox (Knoxville), which rank 3rd and 4th (Office of Comprehensive Health Planning, 1970, p. 30), *all* internships and residencies were located in five high physician ratio counties. It is far more plausible to argue that internships and residencies are concentrated in these counties because of the concentration of practicing physicians there than it is to argue the other way around.

In addition, the faculty must usually be affiliated with a large hospital, and especially a medical-school hospital. In 1971 less than 6 percent of all residency positions in the United States were in hospitals with less than 200 beds, and only slightly more than 1 percent of these were in nonmedical school affiliated hospitals; only 66 percent of the nonaffiliated positions were filled in comparison to 86 percent for the positions in small hospitals with medical school affiliation. For all residency positions regardless of hospital size, 84 percent were in hospitals affiliated with medical schools, 87 percent of which were filled, while 16 percent were in nonaffiliated hospitals, 75 percent of which were filled (American Medical Association 1971). Before a hospital can attract residents, or even before it can even qualify for a residency program, it must be able to attract physicians who can supervise the program. Since a hospital's ability to attract physicians is limited by the social, economic, and demographic potential of the community in which it is located, its ability to develop and implement approved residency programs is also limited by such potential. It is possible, of course, to have medical school affiliated residency programs located in isolated, low-income communities where, because of the linkage with medical schools, adequate faculty supervision could be obtained. Although this would provide a few communities with medical services that residents perform, it would not provide for an increase in the number of permanent physicians in the community. Moreover, such a solution to the maldistribution of physician manpower can have an effect on a very limited number of communities.

The tendency for residents to remain in the locations where they do their residencies, when they in fact do so, may be due to the fact that once a resident physician has completed his residency, he locates in a community that he finds attractive as a place to practice medicine for the same general reasons that other older physicians have found it attractive. In short, practicing physicians are concentrated in certain communities and resident physicians also will tend to concentrate in those communities because of the economic, demographic, and perhaps cultural characteristics of the communities. Note that the five Tennessee counties mentioned above are the first five counties in the median family income and include five of the first eight in population density (persons per square mile) (Anderson county ranks eighth, the other four constitute the first four) (U.S. Bureau of the Census 1967).

In short, things that make settings attractive places for residency programs are also things that make settings attractive for the faculty who supervise residency programs. To introduce residency programs without considering social, economic, and demographic characteristics of the communities in which the programs are located, with the idea that this in itself will lead to the conversion of resident physicians into established practicing physicians, ignores the possibility that the correlation between internship-resident and physician ratios exists because of other conditions. To illustrate, although Tennessee ranked thirteenth in internship-residency positions per 100,000 population in 1968, it still ranked thirtieth in the physician ratio. One factor that is not present in Tennessee's case is a favorable socioeconomic condition, with the state ranking forty-sixth in median family income. Moreover, those areas within the state where residency positions are concentrated are areas of high population density and favorable economic conditions. They are also the areas where physicians are most concentrated.

In general, then, the association between high internship-residency and permanent physician ratios involves several interrelated processes. The location of residency programs depends on the presence of a medical faculty, which normally means a high physician ratio. This, in turn, depends on population size-density, community wealth, and the availability of hospital facilities. These factors may

also influence where a medical school graduate applies for his residency (it may
be the place where he subsequently wishes to establish his practice). There is
little reason, therefore, to expect that the policies which aim to increase the
number of residencies per se will contribute very much toward the solution of a
state's or a community's physician-manpower problem. It will depend on the
characteristics of the places where residency programs are located.

In addition to characteristics of settings in which residency programs are
located, the individual characteristics of the resident may be important. For
example, in the Weiskotten study we do not know whether it is residency position alone or residency position in combination with other factors that leads to
the 63.1 percent figure. It is possible that this relatively high figure attains for
residency because residency is usually combined with one or more other factors,
such as nativity and location of medical school. The results of Donald E. Yett
and Frank A. Sloan (1971) show quite clearly that this *is* the case. In their study
they find that 20 percent of general practitioners who did their internships in a
state other than their native state or where they went to medical school remained
in the state to practice; for specialists and place of residency (instead of internship), the corresponding figure is 16 percent. However, when internship (for
general practitioners) and residency (for specialists) are located in the native
state, the percentages are 75 percent and 58 percent. When internship or residency is in the same state where one attended school, the percentages are 76
percent and 75 percent. Finally, when internships and residencies are located
in the same state in which the individual is a native and attended medical school,
the probability that the physician will establish his initial practice in the state is
0.88 for general practitioners and 0.85 for specialists.

These results are consistent with the conclusions about residency settings.
The association between internship-residency and physician ratios is not a simple matter of internships and residencies being converted into permanent citizens.
Before this happens internships-residencies must be combined with other factors.
Thus, statistically speaking, the effect of internship-residency on where one subsequently practices is a function of the interaction between location of internship-
residency and individual background characteristics, namely nativity and place of
undergraduate medical education.

Therefore, to the extent that residency programs are established for recruitment purposes, such results might suggest that states should recruit for their
internships and residencies those individuals who are state natives, graduates of
state schools, or, preferably, both. Problems are involved here, however.

First, to the extent that background factors should enter into such decisions
is controversial. Traditionally, residents are normally selected primarily because
of their qualifications and not because of their background. To deviate from this
pattern not only raises serious questions about the quality of medicine administered in a particular residency program, it also runs counter to the basic

American value that individuals are to be evaluated on the basis of merit and achievement, not the accidents of birth and fortune, such as the state in which one is born and where he attended school.

But ignoring the value controversy, the results of Yett and Sloan might be taken to indicate that planning should be integrated. One might argue that it is not a question of whether we need more medical schools or more state support for native students in existing state schools or more residency programs. Rather, it is a question of forging linkages between the medical schools and residency programs so that the graduates of the former are feeders for the latter. To create the proper social, educational, and psychological conditions to accomplish this would be no easy matter. Therefore, the success of new residency programs in raising a community's supply of physicians for communities in which residency programs do not now exist can be seriously questioned.

In addition, use of residency programs to recruit physicians to an area may undermine the primary functions of such programs. Since evidence pertaining to the functions of residency programs is extremely limited, comments here must be based largely on logical and theoretical considerations rather than on empirical data. In general, residency programs have been responses to increasing specialization in medicine. As specialization increases, longer periods of post-graduate training are required before physicians are considered by experienced physicians as well qualified to practice particular medical specialties. Granted, residents provide institutions with comparatively cheap physician services and also allow established physicians opportunities to interact with junior colleagues, which can be stimulating experiences, as is the case in all types of graduate education. So, whether intended this way or not, the resident and the institution/ medical faculty supervisors are engaged in an *exchange* from which each derives some benefit. Note that in the evolution of this arrangement residency programs were not designed as recruitment programs. A number of motives no doubt go into the establishment of a residency program (e.g., the need for house staff services, the empire building tendencies of some medical school faculty, etc.), but a viable residency program must provide for some form of exchange. In any case, the traditional medical program has not usually been established in order to recruit more physicians to the state or specific communities. The question arises, therefore: What can be expected of residency programs when they are established specifically to recruit more physicians to a state or community, which appears to be the essence of most proposals linking residency programs to recruitment?

The basis for a viable exchange relationship may be lost. To use residency programs primarily to entice residents to practice in the state or community is likely to lead to faculty behavior that is inconsistent with the kinds of quality learning experiences that most residents seek when they join residency programs. It is possible that medical faculty do things now that make a community or state more attractive to residents, but this is not the kind of behavior that is formally incorporated into a program of postgraduate education very easily (e.g., such as taking time to show residents the *non*medical assets of living in the area).

Thus, the deliberate use of residency programs as recruitment mechanisms is not only controversial in terms of basic values, since criteria other than medical qualifications would be used for purposes of appointment; it may be in conflict with the basic function of post-graduate education. Like any educational program, a residency program can be little better than the quality of the students (that is, residents) in it. Since most physicians capable of and willing to perform faculty roles for residents are probably more interested in the quality of the resident's training than they are in where the resident subsequently locates his practice, the selection of residents will probably continue to be on the basis of the applicant's qualifications, and the primary orientation of the training program will continue to be quality of performance. And if this is not the case, the program is likely to fail, for it will not be attractive to prospective residents; and if it is, it may attract candidates only because they were unable to meet higher standards of other programs.

Conclusion

Programs designed to influence the distribution of physicians by locating more training institutions in areas with physician shortages are not likely to be successful. The same factors that make a community attractive for physicians to practice are also necessary for viable training institutions. Such programs actually may be based on the factual evidence that there is a direct relationship between the number of students (especially interns and residents) per capita of population and the number of practicing physicians per capita. In such instances it is probable that the program is based on an erroneous interpretation of the evidence—that physicians decide to practice in communities where they received their training. A more plausible interpretation is that the number of interns-residents and physicians per capita of population are correlated because each is the result of other conditions, that is, the general social and economic conditions of communities. The success of locating training programs so as to redistribute medical manpower, as well as the actual viability of training institutions, will be constrained by this.

15 Changing Medical Characteristics of Communities

A basic thesis of this book is that many of the causes of the distribution of physicians have a base in general nonmedical differences between communities so that the maldistribution of physicians is in large part the result of processes that lie outside the field of medicine itself. From this it would seem to follow that policy programs should have communities as their focus rather than the individual characteristics of physicians, the national supply and demand, or the location of training institutions, and that effort should be directed to changing medically underserved communities themselves so as to make them more attractive to physicians and to divert more medical resources to them in general. The distinction between medical and general characteristics of communities is relevant in this connection. Changes in the medical characteristics of communities are apt to have a very limited effect on the distribution of physicians. The effects of such changes are constrained by more general community characteristics such as community wealth and population base. In the present chapter two programs are examined from this perspective.

The two programs are the Hill-Burton Construction Program and the Division of Regional Medical Program Service (DRMPS). Both are former federal programs, whose functions are being incorporated into the State Health Planning and Development Agencies for entire States and the Health Systems Agencies for smaller designated geographic regions—Health Service Areas, in accordance with the National Health Planning and Resources Development Act of 1974. Moreover, neither of these programs were oriented specifically to alleviating the maldistribution problem. Nevertheless, both were concerned with effecting changes at the community level. Consequently, an examination of aspects of these programs will highlight some general principles as these relate to the maldistribution problem. It will reveal some of the general difficulties involved when effort is made to redistribute physician manpower and medical services by changing the medical characteristics of communities.

The assessment of both programs is in terms of their effects in one state and one region—Tennessee for Hill-Burton and the Tennessee Mid-South Region for DRMPS. Each program is examined in light of the general framework presented in Chapter 3. They are examined from somewhat different perspectives, however. Hill-Burton is examined with reference to its effect on the distribution of physician manpower, DRMPS with reference to how the distribution of resources by this program has been influenced by the distribution of physician manpower.

Hill-Burton Construction Program

According to statistics published by the American Hospital Association (1967, p. 445; 1970, p. 447), a total of 381,708 beds were established in community hospitals in the United States between 1947 and 1970. A large proportion of these involved federal economic assistance from the Hill-Burton hospital construction program. From the beginning of the program in 1947 to July 1, 1971, the program assisted in the establishment of 344,453 beds in general hospitals (Health Services and Mental Health Administration 1972, p. 21). This is about 90 percent of the beds established in community hospitals during this period. The percentage may be inflated because the time interval is one year longer for figures on Hill-Burton. Discounting this, many beds were no doubt phased out since 1947 (some built with program assistance, some not), making it impossible to know exactly what proportion of all new beds since 1947 involved Hill-Burton assistance. At the same time, the definition of community hospital as used by the American Hospital Association—"nonfederal short-term general or other special hospital whose facilities are available to the entire community" (American Hospital Association 1970, p. 447)—is somewhat broader than the type of hospital to which the Hill-Burton figures refer. There is little doubt, then, that a very substantial proportion of hospital beds established in general community hospitals in the United States since 1947 were established with Hill-Burton assistance. An original objective of this program was to bring about a more even distribution of hospital facilities among communities in the United States. Some evidence suggests that this has been accomplished to a considerable extent, since a disproportionately small share of the funds went to wealthier regions through 1960 (Lerner and Anderson 1963). Closer examination of the effects of the program in one state, Tennessee, questions whether this is to be viewed as a positive consequence.

From 1950 to 1966 a total of 8,355 general hospital beds were financed by the Hill-Burton Program in Tennessee. Since there were 25,137 beds in 1950 and 31,066 in 1967, the number of Hill-Burton financed beds is actually larger than the increase (Tennessee Department of Public Health 1950, p. 6; 1968, pp. 7, 32-33). This apparently is due to some hospitals closing during this period. Since the number of beds involved is unknown, it is not possible to determine what proportion of the total increase was financed by Hill-Burton. It is clear, however, that the proportion is very high. Analysis of the redistribution of general hospital beds by county reveals that the consequences of Hill-Burton did not help the more disadvantaged counties in the state.

First, the r between total Hill-Burton general beds per 1,000 (1960) county population and the 1960 county median family income is 0.17, which does not support the view that Hill-Burton has been particularly successful in assisting the most deprived communities. But it does not support the view that the program was oriented to the most advantaged communities either. Inspection of the data indicates that the distribution of Hill-Burton beds per 100,00 population bears a curvilinear relationship with community wealth. For the 75 counties with the lowest income the correlation is positive and quite low ($r = 0.20$), but for the 20 highest income counties the correlation is negative and moderately high ($r = -0.64$).[a] Inspection of the scatterdiagram indicates a gradual upward trend for the 75 counties in the bottom income range and a rather sharp downward trend for the 20 counties in the upper income range. Thus, up to a certain level Hill-Burton assistance increased slightly as community wealth increased, after which assistance decreased rather sharply as income increased.

A separate issue, however, is whether Hill-Burton led to a *re*distribution of hospital beds. The above analysis reveals only how Hill-Burton beds are distributed, not how the program has (or has not) led to a redistribution of hospital beds, toward a more equal distribution. For this, analysis of changes in the total distribution of beds is necessary. In some counties Hill-Burton beds have been added to existing beds, in others they have been added while some beds have been phased out, and in still others they constitute the only hospital beds in existence. Hence, the relationship between changes in the total hospital-bed ratio at two points in time and community income may be quite different from relationships involving just the Hill-Burton ratio. Consequently, the rate of county change in hospital-bed ratios was computed between 1950 and 1966. Since most general hospital beds added in the state beyond 1949 were added with the assistance of Hill-Burton funds (and facilities supported with Hill-Burton funds were not opened until 1950), most changes in the distribution of hospitals can be attributed to the Hill-Burton Program.

Analysis revealed no relationship whatever between community income and changes in the hospital-bed ratio; $r = 0.00$. Although the relationship of the Hill-Burton ratio and community income is curvilinear, inspection of the scatterdiagram for community income and change in the hospital-bed ratio shows no marked departure from linearity. Hence, the absence of a correlation is not the result of curvilinearity.[b] The program did not eliminate inequities in the availability of hospital beds in this one state.

---

[a]Sources of data: Tennessee Department of Public Health (1950, 1968) and U.S. Bureau of the Census (1967).

[b]The partial correlation between hospital-bed ratio in 1966 and the 1960 county median family income with 1950 hospital-bed ratio controlled yields a correlation of 0.13, slightly higher than the r of 0.00 between income and changes in the ratio. However, because of the curvilinear nature of the relationship between community income and hospital-bed ratio, it is difficult to know how to interpret such results. Therefore, changes in the ratio is used as the method for controlling for the hospital-bed ratios in 1950. The problems associated with such a measure (see Bohrnstedt 1969) are probably less in the present case than those involved with partial correlations when the relationship departs so much from a linear trend.

Hill-Burton and the Redistribution of
Physicians

The central question is whether Hill-Burton influenced the redistribution of physicians in Tennessee counties during the 16-year period. It is still possible that even though Hill-Burton did not altogether help the "worse first" in developing hospital facilities, the communities which needed help most by the program may have been able to attract physicians easier than communities where the need was least. Some have concluded that this indeed has been the case. "Prior to the Hill-Burton program, rural communities and small towns had been at a disadvantage in attracting new physicians. After construction of a modern hospital, rural communities were able to offer recent medical school graduates an attractive field for practice" (Williams and Uzzell 1960, p. 50). The results and interpretations in Chapter 10 suggest quite different expectations.

The overall social and economic resources of a community determine the extent to which it is able to convert existing resources into additional resources. This may significantly influence the outcome of programs of community assistance. S.R. Klatzky (1970) shows, for example, that in spite of the effort by the federal government to equalize the distribution of funds disbursed by the United States Employment Service, the wealthier states get a disproportionately large share of the federal tax funds disbursed by the Service. In a study of the distribution of funds from federal Maternal and Infant Care Project Grants among Standard Metropolitan Statistical Areas and major cities, Judith J. Friedman (1973) finds that projects went disproportionately to areas and cities that had more medical resources (a medical school and a high physician ratio) than areas that had fewer resources (no medical school and a low physician ratio) whereas the tendency for funds to go to areas with especially high need (as indexed by infant mortality rates) was quite weak. In sum, the "impact of [medical] resources . . . is more important than that of need in . . . the distribution of funds" from the maternal and infant care program (Friedman 1973, p. 243).

The process by which the more advantaged communities reap disproportionately greater benefit from federal assistance programs is especially relevant to programs that provide capital resources that are designed to improve human resources in the community (or to upgrade the local occupational-service sector). Niles Hansen (1970) has argued, for example, that federal economic capital programs (e.g., public works programs) for economically depressed regions have not generally led to improvements in the human resources and services of a region—for example, to increases in the number of persons with high level skills and technical expertise—which, in turn, is what leads ultimately to higher personal incomes and increases in the region's overall standard of living. Unfortunately, before such persons are attracted to a community, a strong occupational-service sector must be there to begin with. The extent to which economic and technological increments lead to increases in manpower resources is in direct proportion to the social and economic base in which those increments are introduced.

Hill-Burton is viewed in this context, specifically in terms of the effect of hospital construction on community physician manpower. To this end, the relationship between changes in the physician and hospital-bed ratios between 1950 and 1966 is investigated for Tennessee. Analysis shows that the changes in the two ratios are slightly negatively related ($r = -0.15$). The location of new hospital beds did not follow the movement of physicians over the state, and the movement of physicians was not influenced by any redistribution of hospital beds that may have occurred. To the extent, therefore, that aid in establishing hospital facilities through Hill-Burton was designed at least in part to lead to manpower improvement in communities with a physician shortage—and it would seem hard to argue otherwise, the intended effects did not occur. This is because the potential effects of this program on physician manpower have been modified by the constraints of more general community characteristics. This can be seen from Figure 15-1, which gives the correlation and regression coefficients for median family income and changes in the physician and hospital-bed ratios.[c] During the 1950-66 period, an increase of 3.63 physicians per 100,000 county population was, on the average, associated with a 1960 difference of $1,000 median family income. Comparison of the regression coefficients for the hospital-bed ratios indicates much weaker effects: On the average a county with a 1960 median family income that was $1,000 higher than another county would have increased the number of beds per 100,000 population by less than one bed.[d]

Thus, although changes in the distribution of physicians were patterned on more general county characteristics, this was not true for changes in hospital facilities. Consequently, the Hill-Burton hospital construction program did not lead to a more equitable distribution of physicians in counties in Tennessee. Based on this analysis, therefore, the use of hospital facilities to attract physicians to communities with low physician manpower is not likely to be very successful, and hospital construction programs based on a "worse first" phillosophy are not likely to modify the maldistribution of physicians.

In general, results suggest that programs designed to modify medical characteristics of communities in an effort to attract physicians are not likely to be very successful. This is so because medical characteristics (aside from manpower)

---

[c]Source of data: Source for median family income is U.S. Bureau of the Census (1967). Source for data for hospital beds and physicians are American Hospital Association (1950 and 1967); Maryland Y. Pennell and Marion E. Altenderfer (1954); C.N. Theodore, G.E. Sutter, and E.A. Jokiel (1967). Population figures for 1950 are from U.S. Bureau of the Census (1953) and for 1966 from estimates by the Bureau of Business and Economic Research, University of Tennessee (March 1967).

[d]Correlation coefficients for population density are 0.22 (physicians) and -0.21 (hospital beds) and regression coefficients are 0.0203 and -0.00002. (Recall that when counties have approximately the same number of square miles, population density gives approximately the same values as a measure, such as percentage of urban residents, which combines population size and density.) For the professional ratio, the corresponding correlation coefficients are 0.36 and 0.02 and corresponding regression coefficients are 0.441 and 0.0094.

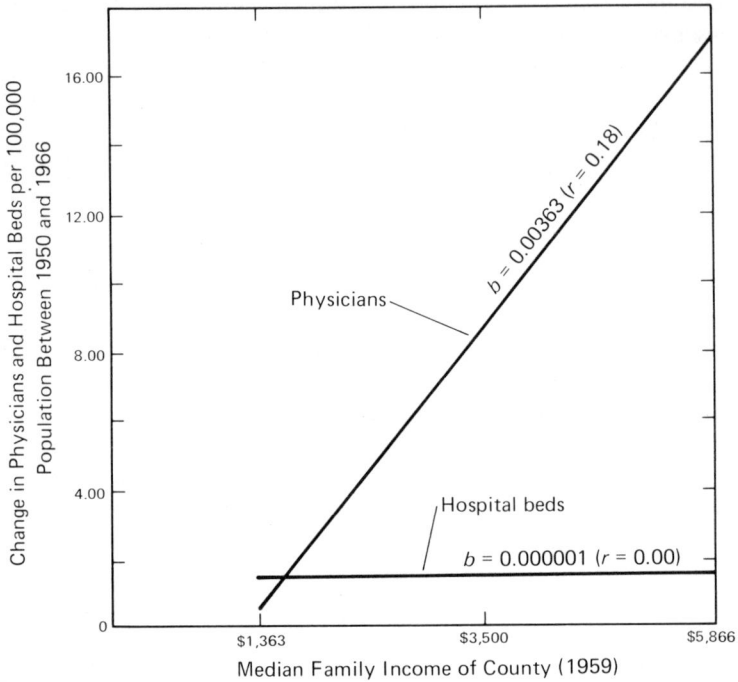

Figure 15-1. Regression of Changes in Physician and Hospital-bed Ratios (1950-66) on Median Family Income (1960) for Tennessee Counties

may be changed with the aid of external funds with no correlative change in phy-sician manpower. The effects of such changes will be modified depending on the general character of the setting in which the changes are introduced. As noted in the first chapter, the establishment of many clinics in underserved communities were of little apparent success in attracting physicians to these communities. Indeed, in many instances the clinics have been converted to nonmedical pur-poses because there are still no physician occupants for them. (See p. 6.)

At the same time, it was seen in Chapter 10 that hospital facilities do influ-ence the distribution of physicians; physicians, especially specialists, are variably attracted to communities depending on their hospital facilities. The same is probably true for free clinics and offices, and similar incentives. It is not improb-able, therefore, that the distribution of physicians would be even worse than it is now if it had not been for the Hill-Burton program and other efforts by com-munities and agencies to attract physicians to underserved communities by establishing medical facilities. This suggests that these programs might be viewed from a somewhat different perspective than is commonly the case. Rather than contending that they have been of substantial benefit to underserved communities or that they have been a waste of effort and money, both perspectives are partially correct. They have not had the benefits that some have claimed; but the distribution of physicians might be considerably more inequitable that it is now if they had not existed.

Regional Medical Program

A federal program for which there were some rather optimistic expectations is the Division of Regional Medical Program Service, which was enacted in law by the 89th Congress (Public Law 89-239). The program has been controversial from the outset; organized medicine has never shown a great deal of enthusiasm for it and medical schools have squabbled over it while at the same time striving to have RMP funds directed their way. Local physicians have not generated a great deal of support for it and many do not understand why it exists. The public, apparently, knows very little about it. Many of the problems associated with this program stem no doubt from the vagueness of the legislation which authorized it, as well as the program's lack of power to generate changes in a system it was supposed to make (Ehrenreich and Ehrenreich 1970). In this section, the relationship between the consequences of this program and the distribution of physician manpower are examined for the Tennessee Mid-South region,[e] for the period 1968-71.

The direction of the Division of Regional Medical Program Service (DRMPS) was to focus on the improvement of medical services for victims and potential victims of "heart disease, cancer, stroke, and related diseases." Attention was directed to the regionwide coordination of services. In 1974 there were 55 RMPs with regions more or less conforming to functional-cultural boundaries, but in many instances confined to, and in other instances influenced by, the political boundaries of the states. In many instances the administrative agency of regional RMPs was a university medical school in the region.

Although program funds were to be dispensed through grants from the federal government, the program was based on a grass roots philosophy. The structure of regional programs was to reflect this. For example, the grant-approving body of Tennessee Mid-South Regional Medical Program (TMS/RMP) was a Regional Advisory Group (RAG), consisting of representatives (medical and nonmedical, but predominantly medical) from communities throughout the region. This group had the responsibility for reviewing all proposals for grant funds and to recommend approval or rejection. These recommendations,

---

[e]As noted in Chapter 13, the area includes 74 counties in middle and east Tennessee (counties lying east of the west transection of the Tennessee River in Tennessee) and 13 counties in southwest Kentucky.

in turn, were usually based on the recommendation of smaller groups (study groups), composed mostly of non-RAG members knowledgeable in the general area (heart, cancer, stroke, continuing education). If approved, the proposal was then submitted to the office of DRMPS in Washington for funding. Moreover, in principle, proposals were to originate at the grass roots level—with individuals from institutions and agencies in local communities, so that the unique problems of particular communities would be reflected in proposal development. As President Johnson stated in his message to Congress on November 8, 1967, "The imagination, knowledge, and energy to operate (the) program will come from the local level." And the intent of the congressional committee that acted on RMP was to "insure local control of programs conducted under the bill." The program, therefore, was theoretically anchored in local communities; the imposition of federal policy on the functioning of local programs was to be minimized. The DRMPS was not to be a planning body so much as an implementing agent.[f]

On the surface, the primary objective of DRMPS would appear to have been organizational—coordination of services on a regionwide basis—rather than distributional, since "the object [was] to influence the present arrangement of health services," with reference to heart disease, cancer, stroke, and related diseases. However, a more equitable distribution was also an aim since "present arrangements" were to be influenced "in a manner that [would] permit the best in modern medical care for heart disease, cancer, stroke, and related diseases to be available to all" (Division of Regional Medical Program 1969). In addition, the emphasis on regionalization implies greater concern for communities and populations not being reached with present methods of health-care delivery.[g] Thus, programs sponsored by TMS/RMP would be expected to be dispersed in communities throughout the region, particularly in light of its grass roots philosophy. Analysis shows, however, that this was not the case in the Tennessee Mid-South region, in large part because of the grass roots philosophy.

---

[f]Some would probably argue that RMPs have been more than anything else *grantor* agencies for awarding federal grants to institutions and communities, and therefore may not differ very much from most other federal granting bodies.

[g]The DRMPS mandate to reorganize and restructure existing medical-care programs is not to be discounted, of course, and is the thing that made the program attractive to many persons. Interestingly, the DRMPS legislation itself makes it extremely difficult to influence reorganization, on a regional or any other basis. This is so because the objective of influencing the "present arrangement of health services" is to be accomplished "without interfering with the patterns, or the methods of financing of patient care of professional practice, or with the administration of hospitals...." And the congressional committee for DRMPS chose "to emphasize that this legislation is intended to be administered in such a way as to make no change whatsoever in the traditional methods of furnishing medical care to patients in the United States, or to financing such care." In essence, the bill states that reorganization is to be achieved without really changing anything and without using those methods that are most likely to be effective in achieving reorganization. See Barbara Ehrenreich and John Ehrenreich (1970).

For this region, Davidson County is second among the counties in median income and median education, third in the ratio of professional workers to total employed labor force, and first in ratio of physicians to population. During the first three years of funding, institutions based in this county got 86 percent of all project grant funds, although only 15 percent of the region's population live in this county.

Since TMS/RMP offices were located in Davidson County, a certain concentration of funds might be expected, regardless of other factors. Moreover, certain programs in Davidson County benefited residents of other counties; for example, personnel from institutions outside Davidson County could obtain additional training through continuing education programs supported by TMS/RMP (e.g., coronary care nursing) and return to their local communities to work. Nevertheless, most of the funds spent in Davidson County went into facilities, services, and programs in medical schools and institutions that primarily benefited individuals who had convenient access to them.[h] (The concentration of funds is reflected in charges by health personnel in other sections of the region that TMS/RMP was primarily interested in programs for Davidson County and the two medical schools.)[i]

Another factor in the concentration of funds is the presence of the region's two medical schools in this county. Others have written about the way local RMPs were dominated by medical schools (Ehrenreich and Ehrenreich 1970). This is at least partially due to medical schools being the sponsoring institutions of many RMPs and are therefore the administrative fiscal agent for them. The influence is not due solely to this, however. Excluding TMS/RMP funds that went to Davidson County, the remaining funds (14 percent of the total) were distributed so that counties with the highest median family income got a disproportionately large share, as the following results reveal (proportion of region's population excluding Davidson County is in parentheses).

Below $3,000	$3,000– $3,499	$3,500– $3,999	$4,000 and over
(25)	(19)	(22)	(34)
11%	14%	36%	40%

---

[h]Over and above any medical advantage, there are economic advantages that accrue to communities which have federally funded medical programs. Hence, not only do such programs contribute to continued inequity in medical care; they also help to extend inequities in the economic realm.

[i]Apparently, the concentration of RMP activity in a few counties is not limited to the Tennessee Mid-South program. For comments on other programs, see "Rating the Regional Medical Plan," *American Medical News* (April 27, 1970), p. 7.

Two explanations for these results can be eliminated. First, the inequitable distribution of funds was not due to attempts by the TMS/RMP staff or the RAG to discriminate against the disadvantaged communities. One of the criteria to be considered in the RAG's evaluation of proposals was community need. Evidence indicates that this helped the communities with physician shortages to some extent. For example, although 82 of 90 proposals were submitted from six counties with more than 100 physicians per 100,000 population (only eight counties have a ratio this high), only 33 percent of these proposals were funded in comparison to 75 percent (six of eight) from the other counties. (For Davidson County, 36 percent were funded.) Second, results are not due to cooptation, in which some antagonistic power group in the environment is incorporated into the organization and, hence, influences the policy of the organization in its own interests (Selznick 1949). There is no evidence that representatives from the affluent communities were brought into TMS/RMP (e.g., through RAG) because they opposed the program or were otherwise antagonistic to it.[j] In any case, this could have had only a minimal effect at most. Although the RAG's approval was crucial, the initiation and development of grant applications was even more so, and members of the RAG were rarely involved at this stage of the process. But, by the same token, increased representation on the RAG of poor communities could have little influence on the distribution of TMS/RMP funds. There had to be a corresponding increase in the development and submission of grant applications from these communities.

Therefore, an explanation more consistent with the facts is that communities were able to attract TMS/RMP resources simply because they had existing manpower resources to attract these resources. Ninety-two percent of the project funds went to three of the eight counties in which the number of physicians per 100,000 population is greater than 100; these counties have only 32 percent of the region's population. Excluding funds that went to Davidson County, 46 percent of the remaining funds went to two counties with physician ratios greater than 1.00, and representing only 19 percent of the remaining population. The distribution of TMS/RMP funds followed the same pattern as the distribution of medical manpower. In general terms, the greater the general wealth of the county, the greater the physician manpower, and hence the greater the county's ability to attract outside financial assistance for medical programs.[k] So long as a

---

[j]It is possible that such a process was at work nevertheless through informal power relations and processes. The author, however, has no reason to believe that these were major factors in the distribution of agency project funds.

[k]In many respects my observations of TMS/RMP are not unlike those reported by the Ehrenreichs (1970) in their analysis of the RMP in New York City. There appear to be more important differences in the two programs, however. In particular, the RAG (and its study groups) was not dominated by the medical schools to the extent that the advisory group appears to have been in New York (although the power of medical schools within TMS/RMP was not an insignificant force, either). But more important is that the TMS

program's funds are allocated through a grant mechanism, and especially when grant proposals are evaluated at least partially on their technical quality, the distribution of funds in favor of communities that need them the least is hard to avoid.

A basic dilemma is posed. On the one hand, it is desirable to support programs that are likely to be successful in providing health care benefits to a target population; but this is most apt to occur where more and better services are already being provided. On the other hand, it is desirable to be fair and to implement the principles of social justice by supporting programs designed to provide health services to disadvantaged populations; but because these are areas where medical manpower is in limited supply, these are precisely those areas where grant applications are not apt to be developed, or if developed, areas with insufficient health care personnel to implement them. In short, these are areas where programs are not likely to be successful.[1]

Conclusion

Neither of the two programs examined in this chapter had as its primary objective the modification of the maldistribution of physician manpower. Certainly DRMPS was not specifically designed to correct for community inequities in physician manpower (although this was certainly not outside it purview), and Hill-Burton was not specifically intended to do this either (although it is hard to imagine that this was not implicit in the program's intent—what good, afterall, are hospital facilities without physicians?). Nevertheless, the two programs have

---

advisory group was not stacked in favor of the medical schools to the extent that it apparently was in the New York program; and in any case, proposals that reached the full TMS/RMP advisory group from study section review were almost always approved. While the forces of power and politics were not absent from TMS/RMP, they alone probably did not result in the inequitable distribution of project funds. At least as important is the nature of the legislation and the structure of the program, which require the utilization of the grant mechanism and which make grant development and implementation dependent on local initiative and resources. These features gave medical schools (and communities where there are more physicians who have the time and ability to write proposals) distinct advantages. Under these circumstances, grantsmanship is power. A major difference between our analysis and the Ehrenreichs' analysis, of course, is that ours is concerned with the distribution of project funds, while the Ehrenreichs' is concerned mostly with the way planning funds were spent (there being only three projects funded in the New York program).

[1]This is not to say that programs in high resource areas and institutions will be successful as judged by the absolute criteria established by the agency from whom grant funds are obtained (such as those of TMS/RMP). But relative to the programs in communities and institutions where resources and personnel are limited—both in quantity and quality, programs where resources and personnel are not so limited are more apt to be successful.

important implications for the maldistribution problem, although the implication is somewhat different in each case.

The distribution of Hill-Burton funds is not correlated with the distribution of physician manpower, and redistribution of hospital facilities over a 16-year period was slightly negatively related to the redistribution of physicians over this period. This was due to the fact that the program was able to influence the distribution of hospital facilities regardless of general social and economic differences between communities, but it was unable to influence the distribution of physician manpower accordingly. The distribution of TMS/RMP resources was a consequence of the uneven distribution of physician manpower. It stemmed from the more advantaged communities having the manpower essential to develop and implement grant applications that, in turn, allowed them to reap the benefits of the program. In spite of different dynamics in each case, the consequences are the same: the effects of the program are modified by the constraints of community structure and inequities are perpetuated or enhanced. In the case of Hill-Burton, the forces of community constraints were overcome to some extent in the distribution of funds for hospital-bed construction. This, however, did not lead to greater equity in the distribution of physician manpower. The use of this and similar programs for dealing with the maldistribution problem is to be questioned.

16

An Alternative Proposal: A Community
and Organizational Perspective

In this book the maldistribution of physicians in United States communities has been examined in an effort to identify significant social and economic factors that contribute to the problem. Focus has been on factors external to medicine. The probable consequences of programs also have been examined in light of the framework and the empirical results concerning those external factors. The general thesis is that the distribution of physicians is deeply rooted in various *non*-medical social and economic conditions of communities and that programs designed to modify the distribution of physicians by making changes in the medical sector will be constrained by these conditions. This is not to say that none of the examined programs will have any positive consequences; all may have beneficial results. Benefits will be quite limited, however, and in some instances they may be realized by only a very few communities. As generalized approaches to the problem, all programs fail to take into account the macrosocioeconomic patterns and processes of which the problem is only one part. The success of all programs will be constrained by this.

In Chapter 12 it was noted that the identification of conditions as "constraints" rather than as "policy variables" does not mean that they should not be given explicit consideration in the development of programs designed to cope with social problems. In this final chapter I will outline a program that is based on the assumption that the success of a program will indeed be constrained by the kinds of community factors that have been shown to be associated with the maldistribution problem. This, of course, will require assumptions as to how these factors will operate in the future. In addition, programs will also be constrained by the future role of the government in alleviating the problem and the future of specialization in medicine.

The Government's Role and What to
Maximize: Community Equity or
Individual Freedom?

A distinction is made between programs that maximize physicians' autonomy (or that preserve physicians' autonomy intact) and programs that would reduce their autonomy. The value of a more equable distribution of physicians may not be the only, or perhaps even the most important, value to consider. The freedom of individuals to choose the communities in which they live and work is also important. At issue here is the question: Can solutions to the problem of extreme community inequity in physician manpower be met within a social framework that permits health professionals a free choice in selecting their community of residence? For the nation to realize the objective of equitable health services, to which it appears to be committed, constraints on the movement of health professionals may be considered necessary. Although legislation has not been passed that would coerce physicians to live in some communities rather than others, such legislation is by no means inconceivable. Indeed, physicians and nonphysicians alike have advanced the proposition to the author that graduates of medical schools should be required to spend a portion of their postgraduate years practicing medicine in communities where physician manpower is in short supply. Such programs might solve the problem of community inequity, at the expense of autonomy and freedom for individual health professionals. But for the the government of a free society to impose such constraints on individuals would be distasteful for some of those who impose them. Moreover, if the government can do this for one occupation, why can't it do it for other occupations—engineers, lawyers, teachers, social workers, nurses, and so forth?[a] Many will agree that the consequences of such a policy would probably be more undesirable than those the policy is designed to eliminate. At the same time, we are faced with the question raised a number of years ago: "Can the undirected forces in a free society be relied upon to effect an equable distribution of physicians?" (Mountin, Pennell, and Nicolay 1942a, p. 1373). As we have seen throughout this book, the undirected forces of our society are certainly not moving in such a direction; and evidence indicates that this has been the case for some time now. Moreover, with the emergence of suburbs, inner cities have joined low-income, rural communities as places with physician shortages. Viewed from this perspective alone, an answer to the above question would seem to be negative. A more equable distribution of physicians in communities in the country would not appear feasible in the absence of constraints on where physicians choose to live and work.

The issue here is part of a broader conflict between individual autonomy and equality of opportunity. To guarantee that opportunities are more equal, the courts and federal government have had to impose constraints on how some individuals, businesses, and communities conduct their affairs. The conflict over school bussing, which is intended to promote racial school integration and,

---

[a]There is the argument that because the public pays such a high proportion of all medical education—student tuition covers only a small part—different circumstances exist in the case of the medical profession. There is an element of truth here, but it is subject to question because virtually no class of students pays for all its education through tuition. In addition, unlike other professionals, most physicians devote a considerable period of time—from one to several years—in internships and residencies for a relatively low salary. Consequently, one might argue that the medical professional, more than other professional, repays society for the support he/she has received in training.

therefore, greater equality of educational opportunity between races, is a recent example. Many individuals and communities feel that court-ordered bussing is an infringement on their freedom to control a local institution. At least for the foreseeable future the use of government constraints to enhance equality of opportunity at the expense of individual and community autonomy may have run its course: It is not a good thing to do from a political standpoint. Consequently, it is probably safe to assume that the government will not attempt to restrict physicians' freedom to select their community of practice.[b] The redistribution of physicians in the future will probably have to come some other way.

Future of Specialization

We have seen that level of specialization is related directly to community structure. This pattern is interpreted in terms of physicians' occupational opportunity: Physicians gravitate to environments that will provide them with the most opportunities to do what they have been trained to do. According to this interpretation, added remuneration or special compensation (e.g., free clinics) will probably not be sufficient to attract physicians to most communities with low physician manpower. Such programs are based on a false premise, and this is that the primary motivation of most physicians in establishing their community of residence is economic rather than occupational opportunity. The distinction is a fine one, but important. By occupational opportunity I mean the opportunity for an individual to perform the type of job he has been trained to do and that he wishes to perform. While this involves economic motivation,

---

[b]The assumption is subject to question. Efforts have been made in the U.S. Congress to introduce health manpower legislation that would make service in physician shortage areas mandatory for a number of physicians. It is not clear at this time that such legislation will pass (it has been met with opposition by some members of Congress) or exactly what form it will take. Traditional approaches have tried to obligate physician students to service in underserved areas through the provision of student loans that may be excused upon completion of service in an underserved area. This approach has frequently failed because once graduated, individuals choose to pay the loan back in money rather than service. Another proposal before Congress, but not passed, is a program of aid for medical schools based on the number of students enrolled, but contingent on all of its students signing an agreement with the government to serve for two years in underserved populations if needed. This would be a rather serious intrusion on the autonomy of individual medical professionals—and it pressures medical schools, in return for federal monetary support, to require something of their students that members of Congress may not wish to impose. In any case, such legislation would probably not contribute very much to alleviating the maldistribution of physicians; underserved communities would still not receive medical care on a permanent and continuous basis, since physicians would be obligated for only a period of two years. It is probable that the primary consequence of such half-hearted mandatory service approaches will only restrict, and endanger for the future, the freedom of medical professionals without having a significant positive effect on the maldistribution problem.

economic motive is not the sole (or even the primary) factor involved in choosing one community of residence over another. It is probable that many
specialists currently practicing in populous affluent areas could make as much
money working as general practitioners in less populous and less affluent communities. In any case, let us assume that many specialists could function as
general practitioners. It is not likely, however, that many want to be general
practitioners regardless of the income they might receive in any type of environment. Most probably prefer to do what they have been trained to do, and will
therefore locate in environments that will permit them to do this.

If this distinction between economic and occupational opportunity motivation is valid, changes in the products of medical schools could influence the
distribution of physicians considerably. Specifically, training more generalists
and fewer specialists would provide a larger number of physicians who would
be able to find opportunities to practice their trade in communities currently
characterized by low physician manpower. But as was seen in Chapter 12, the
effects would be limited unless the number of student-physicians from underserved areas increased. Also, a decrease in specialization is doubtful. Given the
existing technological and knowledge base of medicine, it is probable that
specialization will actually increase in the future. Some authors have even suggested that we may see the development of superspecialists, beyond what we
have called limited specialists (Field 1970). Given the current trend, in a few
years general practice and even family medicine may be a thing of the past.
There would, of course, be negative consequences of this. Problems of coordi-
nating patient care, which were discussed in Chapter 11, as well as increases in
the impersonality and fragmentation of patient care would be the likely result.
But all consequences of the trend would not be negative; and on balance, the
demise of the general practitioner and the increase in specialization may be
positive. Better treatments of diseases that cripple and kill (e.g., cancer, diabetes,
heart disease, and stroke) may be possible. Therefore, care may become more
impersonal and less continuous, but technically of a higher quality. "Despite
certain evils of specialization which have received a good deal of attention in
recent years, we believe that the growth of specialization has been a more important factor in improving the quality of medical care" (Terris and Monk 1956,
p. 588). But the relative benefits and liabilities of specialization aside, a continued increase in specialization probably can be expected and will be a force
that will make it difficult to modify the current maldistribution of physicians.

Community and the Future

Before discussing what the dominant socioeconomic trends of the future
are likely to be, it will be worthwhile to distinguish between two kinds of programs designed to modify the distribution of physicians. Some, such as those

reviewed in the previous four chapters focus exclusively on aspects of the medical institution. A limitation of all such programs is that they are not integrated with the forces that have contributed to the problem in the first place. Indeed, in some instances, such as Hill-Burton and proposals to locate training institutions in underserved areas, programs actually run counter to those forces. And, if the thesis and analysis in this book are valid, such programs will not succeed in resolving the basic problem (indeed, they may make it worse) because they run counter to social and economic forces over which the programs have virtually no control. It is the difference between communities in general social and economic factors that is the crucial problem and programs directed only to aspects of the medical institution contribute very slightly if at all to reducing these more general differences.

This conclusion may suggest an approach that focuses on the total social and economic revitalization of rural and economically depressed communities and the inner cities. Many federal programs concerned with rural poverty have been based on the premise that it is desirable and possible to revitalize the economic and social institutions of disadvantaged communities. In the Agricultural Act of 1970, Congress declared, "The highest priority must be given to the revitalization and development of rural areas." Since the distribution of physicians is patterned on general differences between communities and is, in fact, just one aspect of those differences, the social and economic growth of deprived communities would, according to the framework of this book, contribute to the solution of physician manpower inequalities between communities.

The framework in Chapter 3 does not lead to optimism, however. Overall revitalization requires the development of an economic sector, population base, and local service sector. The way these aspects of community are linked does not encourage optimism that programs designed to revitalize the social and economic institutions of disadvantaged communities will be very successful. Locational patterns in industry require a certain population base, as well as a strong local service sector and high-level occupational skill mix, which are themselves also consequences of industrial concentration. And as Wilbur P. Thompson (1969) notes, the industries that do relocate in disadvantaged communities tend not to increase the community's relative socioeconomic position because it is the slow growing, dieing, and low-paying industries that move to such communities. And Niles M. Hansen (1970) notes that attempts to strengthen the local service sector and raise the occupational skill mix of economically depressed communities are most apt to result in the out-migration of individuals who have received occupational and academic training that qualifies them for economically lucrative jobs. To try to reverse these patterns would require that fast-growing and high-skill industries would have to locate in areas where the labor force is deficient in numbers and in skill requirements. This would not only create problems for the industries themselves, it would also create massive problems of occupational and industrial dislocation in areas now characterized by social and economic advantages. It would establish industries in settings where external economies do not exist and where the necessary environmental supports, such as population, labor skill, and professional services—all of which are requirements of an industrial community, simply do exist.[c] Such efforts would be expensive, and they would be inefficient. They would also run counter to historic socioeconomic trends in society.

But will these trends hold true in the future? I think a realistic assessment yields an affirmative answer. Thompson views the growth of community as resembling a growth loop between industrial development at one end and population growth at the other. Intervening between the two are changes in industry mix, sophistication and variety of the labor skills, increases in income, and upgrading of the local service sector along with more and wider range of services, including the high services such as medicine. Community growth, once started, tends to perpetuate itself. "We move from the local industry mix to the rate of local growth in employment and population, and then . . . growing size feeds back to restructure the local economy so as to virtually ensure further growth" (Thompson 1969, p. 3).

Still, the argument that industries can be attracted to economically depressed communities and regions of the country finds support. Indeed, according to Hansen, "the regional policy in the United States has been formulated and implemented on the assumption that it is possible to attract sufficient industry to lagging, and for the most part rural, regions of the country to give residents of these regions economic opportunities comparable to those enjoyed by other Americans" (Hansen 1970, p. 298). Programs, for example, Appalachian Regional Development Act of 1965, are passed by Congress "on the assumption that sufficient economic activity [can] be attracted to the region to give it a high and sustained rate of economic growth, and that employment opportunities approaching those in the rest of the nation [can] be achieved without significant outmigration" (Hansen 1970, p. 292). Hansen (1970) contends, however, that such programs have not been successful. To attract industries a community must provide for external economies, and external economies are linked to urban (or population) growth. Even when lagging

---

[c]The problem here is not unlike the problem of development in underdeveloped countries. Debate continues as to the best way to develop such contries. Some emphasize capital, others skill and education, and others culture, social structure, and political institutions. Since these factors are interrelated, a problem is where to start and how the overall society can be changed by introducing changes in only one part. Bert F. Hoselitz states: "If advancing and stagnating economies (societies) are contrasted with one another, the crucial question immediately arises as to what factors determine the point of 'take off.' This is merely another way of asking what factors differentiate advancing from stagnant economies and is equivalent to pointing to the practical policy problem of what changes must be made in stagnating economies in order to push them to a level of output where self-sustained groups will begin" (Hoselitz 1967, p. 271). The statement can be applied to the economically advancing and stagnating communities within society.

regions and communities are able to attract industry, the area may still lag behind because of the kind of industry the area is likely to attract.

Processes that have made for general social and economic differences between communities in the past will tend to do so in the future. Hence, programs of over-all economic development for communities will not work in solving the problems of community poverty. Consequently, we are apt to see a continuation of cur-rent trends rather than the revitalization of rural economically depressed areas (although these may occur in isolated instances, depending on happenstance and good fortune—for example, discovery of mineral deposits). The future will be dominated by growth centers, rather than a large number of small disadvantaged communities suddenly developing industrial and economic muscle. And since industrial development, population growth, skill mix, community wealth, and the service sector are all part of the same general process, physicians can be expected to continue concentrating in some communities and avoiding others. The trend toward concentration is characteristic of the service industry as well as the manu-facturing industry, and according to Thompson it is more so. This stems from the role of access in locational patterns. Moreover, the high services, including medicine, may play a leading role in this increased concentration. A quote from Thompson in Chapter 2 may be elaborated.

> The declining role of land and the rising role of access . . . acts to rein-force the advantage of the larger urban area in the competitive struggle for industry. While the trend to market orientation may well have been up to now largely a result of the shift in emphasis from material proces-sing to product fabricating within manufacturing, the locational power of the mass market may in coming decades rest more on the coming dominance of the high services. Extractive industries gain from being dispersed to avoid the diminishing returns of very intensive cultivation or extraction, while manufacturing operations, and services even more, seem to experience a rather long state of increasing returns with higher densities. Manufacturing at a large scale requires the assembling of large work forces, and the movement of persons (job commuting) is, on the whole, much more expensive that the transportation of material or prod-uct. But service industries need to weigh the costs of movement of both the producer (lawyer, doctor, teacher) and the consumer (client, patient, student), although these are sometimes substitutive (the house-call). A dense cluster of people—a city—is almost by definition a physi-cal manifestation of a planned arrangement for the heavy physical interaction especially characteristics of the service industries (Thompson 1969, p. 12).

According to this analysis, then, "one gets a very strong feeling of near-inexorable urban growth through the population range from 200,000 to 16 million . . . . The argument is, in sum, that metropolitan areas of a million and over develop industrial instructures especially suited to give birth to *new industries,* and they amass markets especially attractive to the *income-elastic high services.* With possession of both kinds of high-growth industries, it will be extremely difficult to restrain their growth, and it is far from clear that we should even try to do so" (Thompson 1969, p. 12; author's emphasis). Hence, the distribution of physicians will continue to be only one facet of a macro-socioeconomic process involving the distribution of new industries, occupational skills, population wealth, and high services. The processes through which communities gain advantages over others is difficult to modify, and for the country as a whole it is probably not even possible.

Is There an Alternative?

According to this analysis, then, both the dominant trends in medicine (specialization) and society are working toward maintaining the present maldistribution of physicians or of making it worse. Programs directed to aspects of the medical institution alone yield few positive results, and attempts to modify socioeconomic forces through the revitalization of disadvantaged communities are probably futile. A more realistic strategy would strike a balance between the extreme approaches of trying to influence the distribution of physicians by trying to manipulate aspects of the medical institution or of trying to modify the array of social and economic forces that are causal in the distributional problem. At the same time, such a plan should safeguard the autonomy of the individual's choice of residence as well as provide for greater equity in the distribution of physician services.

Results have shown that the physician shortage characterizes two different types of communities—economically depressed rural counties and inner cities. Results have also suggested that the nature of the problem is somewhat different for the two types of communities. The shortage of specialists is much greater than the shortage of generalists in the low income, rural places, whereas in large cities the shortage of generalists and other primary-care providers seems to be more critical. The problem for underserved low-income, rural areas will be considered first.

If it is true that one reason specialists tend to concentrate in populous dense areas is because they are apt to find greater occupational opportunity there, a strategy is suggested. Ignoring the question of community wealth and cultural attraction for the moment, if guarantees could be given to specialists that there would be a sufficient demand for their special skills in sparsely populated areas, they might be attracted to such areas. This would mean that the population to be served would have to extend beyond the boundaries of a particular community. The establishment of greater intercommunity medical relationships and referral systems among physicians might be one method by which the critical mass necessary for specialty practice is achieved. This strategy should also recognize that specialists are more apt to be attracted to wealthier communities. Effort should be made to recruit for communities where the economic, social and cultural advantages are not so low. Several sparsley populated counties could then be combined with such a county to form an "intercommunity medical network."

In addition, the establishment of medical facilities in the central county may make the arrangement even more appealing. We have seen that the effect of the hospital-bed ratio on the specialist ratio is greater under conditions of high size-density and high income. By substituting an extended catchment area for the local population base, it is possible to combine the three factors that are important in attracting specialist physicians to a community—population base (size-density), community wealth, and specialized facilities.

Attemps could be made, therefore, to establish intercommunity systems of referral. Configurations of counties in various parts of the country could be identified on the basis of total population, and where possible, a county with at least moderately high economic development should be selected as the place where specialists might be concentrated. And this is not to say that the community must be a large metropolitan area. The actual community selected as the focus would depend also on its potential for developing relationships with other communities, which represented a combined population base that would be large enough to attract additional specialists. The recommendation is, thus, to join a systematization of the medical referral system with a recruitment program. In addition, support for additional medical-technical facilities could be given to those communities where it is less difficult to recruit specialists. Such support is especially recommended in light of the observation that hospitals appear to be emerging as functional alternatives for solo general practitioners in the referral process, especially with reference to limited specialists. Consequently, effort might be made to have the hospital in the central community the focal point of the intercommunity medical network. Ideally, the hospital would be given the responsibility for assuring that citizens in the designated network receive medical care, either through physicians associated with the hospital itself or through satellite centers in outlying communities. Although this will provide for greater continuity of care—patient medical records will be centralized to a greater extent than is now the case, it will also lead to more impersonal care which tends to accompany all forms of institutionalized care. But this is already occurring and is probably inevitable, and not just in medicine. "It is likely that many long-term social trends will continue into the 1990's"; and included in these trends is the increased trend toward bureaucratization (Jacoby 1973, p. 252). The advantage of making the hospital the center, aside from the fact that it appears to be emerging as the center of medical care anyway, is that it allows for the concentration of responsibility. With the locus of responsibility in an organizational setting, individual members of the organization can be constrained to act in accordance with organizational requirements. Specifically, medical staff would be required, as members of the hospital staff, to assist in the development, implementation and continued operation of the intercommunity network. Without having an organizational base for such a program, the alternative is to convince large numbers of physicians individually that they should shift their allegiance from the particular patients in the community to the entire community, or more properly in this case, to several communities. The difficulties in this alternative are obvious; and they are probably insurmountable.

This is not to say that all physicians should become salaried hospital physicians. Some may be, but it is not necessary to the program of action being suggested. The only requirement is that physicians adapt their behavior to the requirements of the institution that provides them with facilities and personnel to care for their patients. Whether they are paid in salary or in fees is not a crucial issue.

Many physicians no doubt would openly resist such a program. And there is the additional problem of how to get medical organizations, such as hospitals, and especially the physician members of them, to assume responsibility for the health care of several communities, or even of one entire community for that matter. Such resistance could be neutralized, however, if hospital certification and funds were contingent on the hospital extending its reach to depressed communities, and it were made clear that physician hospital privileges were contingent on their participation in the plan. Moreover, with federal or state assistance, some hospitals could be upgraded and facilities extended, thus making them more attractive to physician specialists. This would be further inducement for physician cooperation. Such upgrading and extension of facilities would not necessarily occur in communities where hospitals were of poor quality or where physician manpower is in short supply. Rather, it would occur in communities that are strategically located so that it would be the center of an intercommunity medical network. In many instances hospitals would already be of good quality and physician manpower would be adequate for local community needs. Additional resources would be provided so the hospital and the physicians associated with it could extend services to a wider population. And as the number of patients increased, that is, as the demand for medical care increased, an increase in the supply of physicians could be expected.

Finally, there is the question of financial mechanisms and mode of payment. Different alternatives are possible. In some networks, some form of prepaid capitation plan might be best; the hospital would be responsible for seeing that all members of a designated area receive medical care for an annual fee per capita. There are several drawbacks to such a plan. An exact listing of persons in the population would have to be kept, as would a record of individuals who migrate in and out of the several communities. Another possible drawback is that hospitals might attempt to extend or contract their intercommunity networks primarily for financial reasons rather than to reduce the inequalities in community access. Also, a capitation plan might require a larger number of salaried physicians than there are physicians who prefer this form of remuneration. A fee for service plan would probably provide greater flexibility and reduce a considerable amount of record keeping and administrative detail. It would allow physicians to retain their own offices if they wished, as long as their medical records were centralized. It would leave more alternatives open to the patient; he could choose another hospital and physicians outside the network without having to sacrifice the prepaid capitation fee that has already been paid.

In summary, it is suggested that intercommunity medical networks be established around a community that, because of its social and economic resources, and in combination with the population of surrounding communities, could support a viable medical community. Hospital facilities would be upgraded and extended in return for the hospital staff assuming responsibility for providing care to a wider population. Physicians would be responsible for developing and implementing such a plan in return for continued access to hospital facilities. Referral systems would be developed, or systematized where they now exist, between physicians in the central community and physicians in outlying communities.

There are several advantages to such a program. First of all, it does not work against social and economic constraints imposed by the social structure. Indeed, it recognizes that processes generated by differences between communities and population concentration cannot be reversed by administrative, political, or medical action. The plan would call for a form of reorganization that is adapted to the broader environment of which such organization is a part. Organizations that are not well adapted to their environment are not apt to survive, and certainly they won't be effective.

The introduction of formal organization almost inevitably imposes constraints on the participants in the organization. The current case is no exception; some physicians would have less autonomy than they have now. At the same time, the constraints would be minimal; physician autonomy would not be seriously threatened despite a change in the system. Physicians need not relinquish their responsibility and commitment to specific patients. Indeed, the development of systematic referral networks, even with the hospital as the center, does not interfere with the particularized relationships between physicians and patients at all. A physician's patients would just come from a wider range of communities. Actually, no basically new elements would be introduced into the medical system at all. All that may be new is the rationalization and systematization of a process that already exists to some extent.[d]

---

[d]For example, in a continuous daily survey covering a 27-month period in two economically depressed counties in southern Appalachia with low physician ratios, individuals were asked if they or members of their household had visited a physician within two weeks of the

Consequently, physicians should experience little difficulty in adapting to the new system since the range and scope of behaviors to be changed are limited.

To the extent that such a strategy were successful, it would reduce pressures on physicians in isolated and disadvantaged communities. A systematically organized referral system would be more or less accessible to them. And the fact that patients will be aware of this would create pressure on generalists to refer patients for appropriate specialized care. Better quality of care should result. And a reduction of physician work pressure would give the physician more leisure, provide more opportunities for continuing education, and hopefully, would slow the exodus of physicians from underserved communities.

Although additional hospital facilities would be necessary, the implementation of the proposed strategy would be more economical than most other programs designed to redress the distributional problem. Many hospitals in smaller communities could be phased out, although in some instances they might be retained as satellite centers. Economies are achieved primarily because the program is designed to increase access (and probably it will lead to improved quality as well) with existing manpower, although it does not preclude the incorporation of various paramedical personnel, such as physician's assistants. Changes that occur have to do only with the way physicians are arranged in reference to the process by which they refer and receive patients, and even here the change would probably not be a major modification from the existing system.

Different communities and sets of communities have problems that differ from others, of course. A program such as that advocated here may not be tailored to meet the most pressing needs of some areas. At the same time, however, it would be sufficiently flexible that it could be adapted to the peculiarities of specific areas and is not inconsistent with programs geared to meet unique problems of individual communities and areas. It could be integrated with a large number of programs. It would, of course, run counter to programs that are designed to increase the medical facilities and manpower in communities which do not have sufficient social and economic resources to support them.

Even so, community inequities in medical care would continue to exist. In many communities the availability of medical care will be less than in socially and economically advantaged communities. Members of many communities will still be inconvenienced by not having the appropriate medical care locally available. In addition, the success of such a program would not be quick or dramatic.

---

interview and whether the visit were in or outside the county. Over 16,000 individuals are represented from the two counties. Of those who has seen a physician, 40.5 percent went outside the county. And of those who were hospitalized, 49.4 percent were hospitalized outside their home county (each county has its own hospital). These findings are reported by Miles and Rushing (1975).

A period of years would probably be necessary before any effect could be detected. And there are other problems.

First, even assuming the implementation of these recommendations, there is the problem of where to start. Systems of referral cannot be systematized until a sufficient number of appropriate specialists are available. At the same time, it is the system of referrals (and the wider catchment area) that will probably attract specialists. This is a chicken and egg problem. At the same time, once started, the process should be self-perpetuating. That is, a systematic intercommunity referral system will attract specialists, and the availability of specialists should increase the utilization of the system. In the beginning, a program of recruitment should accompany efforts to systematize intercommunity referral systems.

Second, more knowledge of existing referral patterns and practices in particular areas would probably be needed before specific programs were put into effect. Physician referrals are probably based on a number of factors—friendship, status, reciprocity, and prejudice and not just what is best for the patient, medically and financially (Shortell 1973, 1974). This is probably true both with reference to the community to which a patient may be referred, as well as the specific physician. Some resistance to a referral system that is designed to improve the medical care of a configuration of communities can therefore be expected. It is probable that research on the way referrals are made in specific areas would be necessary before optimum results could be expected. Where possible, there should be as little disturbance in the present system as possible. Intercommunity likes and dislikes might be criteria to consider in arranging communities into intercommunity referral systems.

Third, the structure of the proposed program does not require that individual physicians identify with or assume responsibility for a configuration of communities, or even their own community as fully as some might wish. It allows the physician to remain individually responsible only to particular patients who come to him for service. While this may not be desirable in itself, the fact that it is a deeply institutionalized pattern of American medicine indicates that any attempt to change it will encounter severe resistance. (This is not to say that efforts should not be made to modify this pattern. However, it probably should not be an explicit part of a program designed to attract physicians to areas of low manpower by developing intercommunity referral systems.)

Fourth, although examination of existing data may permit the identification of several clusters of communities, with one of them possessing significant socioeconomic advantages, it will not always be possible to combine such communities into an integrated network because of geographical and other barriers that separate them.

The type of program suggested is not new. Others have advocated somewhat similar programs (cf. Rutstein 1967; McNerney and Riedel 1962). The proposed line of action is not unlike medical clinics and centers, such as the Drover Clinic in Madisonville, Kentucky, which are already providing health care for several communities on a systematic basis. The Area Health Education Program, which provides for medical school-linked community centers of continuing education for practicing physicians, is an emerging development that appears to be consistent with the above. The comprehensive National Health Planning and Resources Development Act of 1974 is especially consistent with the proposal. This Act authorizes the establishment of State Health Planning and Development Agencies for planning health services on a statewide basis and Health Systems Agencies for planning within smaller geographic areas, known as "health service areas." Agencies are to develop plans for the health care for populations in rural and economically depressed areas and create institutions that will "provide various levels of care (including intensive care, acute general care, and extended care) on a geographically integrated basis." The overall function of the Health Service Agency is to develop a geographically coordinated plan of health services that would insure that all persons in the area have access to the type of care needed at reasonable cost and at the same time prevent unnecessary duplication of health resources. With appropriate authority Health System Agencies could provide the administrative structure within which the program suggested here could be implemented on a systematic basis.

Finally, in its emphasis, the type of program advocated departs somewhat from the traditional emphasis of so many other plans to provide health care to underserved populations. This is that attention focuses more on secondary care than on primary care. For many communities in the United States the delivery of primary care is becoming an increasingly difficult matter because providers of primary care are not locally available. Although this may not be a desirable trend, it is not likely to change just because many believe that the demise of primary care physicians in disadvantaged communities (and increasingly in advantaged communities as well, at least relative to specialists) is undesirable. Programs designed to link disadvantaged communities to systematic referral networks that bring persons with medical needs to settings in which specialty care as well as primary care, but especially specialty care, is available is a more plausible approach.

Programs for underserved areas in large urban places would contain some of the same features as programs for underserved rural areas, although there would be differences. As above, the responsibility for assuring that certain underserved populations receive medical care would be delegated to a hospital (or other medical organization). In return for the use of hospital facilities, physicians would be responsible for assuring that the appropriate levels and types of care were available for the population. This would have to be accompanied by a stringent policy of regional planning agencies and certification and licensing bodies to prevent the construction and expansion of hospital facilities in surburban communities that might attract specialty physicians away from the city hospitals. The problem of suburbs attracting generalists and even general specialists might continue, as results in Chapter 9 would suggest. This problem might be somewhat alleviated provided medical schools are successful in training a larger number of family practitioners. However, this particular problem will probably remain until the social composition of cities begins to change. The types of physician-patient relationships that are especially desirable in primary care may be difficult to obtain for inner-city residents until the process of suburbanization has stopped. At the same time, universal health insurance may persuade primary-care physicians to locate their practices near hospitals in the inner city even if they chose to live outside the city. It may be necessary to allocate the responsibility of care for underserved populations in the inner city to hospitals in the surrounding suburbs, and physicians using those hospitals would be required to see that the appropriate types of treatment were made available. Solutions to the shortage of primary care in the cities may be harder to effect than solutions of specialty care for rural populations. In both instances, however, responsibility for care would be lodged with hospitals or other medical organizations, and in return for their use of facilities in those organizations physicians would be required to devise programs that assured that the medical needs of underserved populations were met. This obviously means that the mission of hospitals would change—they would have less freedom of location and construction of facilities than they have had in the past, and physicians would have to be more responsive to the mission of hospitals. Such changes would have to be supported by regional planning bodies with the authority to assure that their plans were implemented. This, of course, imposes constraints on the degree of freedom possessed by health-care providers. But these would be less constraining than the policies which direct individuals where they could live and work.[e]

Conclusion

The distribution of physicians in the United States has been examined with a specific effort to account for differences in physician manpower between communities. A line of action has been proposed that would appear to have more promise of success than a number of alternatives that have been examined. The proposal recognizes that programs that focus exclusively on the medical institution are likely to have very limited results. It also recognizes that the maldistribution of physicians—or almost any social problem, for that matter—cannot be solved merely through administrative actions and government regulations and statutes. This is so because such actions, regulations, and statutes—state manipulation—do not modify the socioeconomic context of communities,

---

[e]Reference here is to proposed legislation that would require mandatory service for a period of time in underserved areas.

out of which the problem emerges.[f] And while it recognizes that the medical institution, and specifically the maldistribution of physicians, is only part of a broader pattern, the proposal does not recommend the modification of the broader pattern—which would be unrealistic. Instead, the proposal urges the affiliation of disadvantaged communities with advantaged communities so that the medical needs of the members of the former can be met more adequately. More than that, it recognizes that the establishment of such intercommunity networks will lead to a wider range of medical services for communities which already enjoy socioeconomic advantages by making such communities even more attractive to physicians, particularly to specialists, which in turn will have a reciprocal effect on the more disadvantaged communities, and so forth. From the standpoint of medical services, networks of communities are possible in which the amount and range of medical services in the advantaged and disadvantaged communities are mutually dependent. Gain for one will not be at the expense of the other. At the same time, in directing its efforts to the problem of insufficient medical resources of disadvantaged communities, the proposal is not doomed to almost inevitable failure because of the socioeconomic constraints of society.

At the same time, it is not argued that programs directed specifically at changing various aspects of the medical institution would yield no benefit, or that the type of program outlined here precludes some of the programs that have been suggested. On the contrary, the integration of some of these programs, such as training more general and family practitioners and physicians assistants, with a program similar to that outlined here would contribute to the strength of those programs. The different programs would serve to complement each other and, together, would probably yield greater benefit toward solving the maldistribution problem than either one by itself. Programs designed to increase general and family practitioners and train more physician assistants, by themselves, fail to recognize that for these types of workers to have their maximum

---

[f]Some will probably view such a program of action as too conservative. But I suspect that to the extent that any social problem has its roots in the structure of society, any successful solution must proceed somewhat cautiously and be adapted to the causal forces creating the problem. Usually public policy actions are artificial in the sense that they are not true emergents from the structure of society. The approach here is more aptly characterized as realistic than as conservative. Indeed, many programs that are based on the rather simple notion that problems can be solved through mere government manipulation are really quite conservative simply because they do not change anything. I am reminded of a quote that is more than 70 years old, by the famous French sociologist Emile Durkheim. In commenting on his view of society, he stated: "We are even, in a sense, essentially conservative, since we deal with social facts as such, recognize their flexibility, but conceive them as deterministic rather than arbitrary. How much more dangerous is the doctrine which sees in social phenomena only the results of unrestrained manipulation, which can in an instant, by a simple dialectical artifice, be completely upset!" (Durkheim 1937, p. xxxix). American public policy too often has been based on such a doctrine.

effect, some form of community and organizational support may be necessary. Since I view community inequity in physician manpower as interrelated with other aspects of the American social structure and as a reflection of that structure, the problem is not considered merely or even primarily one of numbers. In commenting on the medical crisis, the National Advisory Commission on Health Manpower stated (1967, Vol. 1, p. 2):

> The crisis . . . is not simply one of numbers. It is true that substantially increased numbers of health manpower will be needed over time. But if additional personnel are employed in the present manner and within the present patterns and "systems" of care, they will not avert, or even perhaps alleviate, the crisis. Unless we improve the system through which health care is provided, care will continue to become unsatisfactory . . .

I have extended the argument. Disadvantaged communities are not likely to undergo a social and economic revolution that in time will contribute to a solution of medical care in such communities. I believe, instead, that socially and economically depressed communities will continue to be depressed in the future, regardless of efforts made by the government to change their situations. The contention is that the distribution of physician manpower is a result of general social and economic differences between communities. It would follow, then, that an increase in available health care for citizens in communities where manpower and facilities are lacking, or in short supply, will not come about through an increase in numbers alone, but through some form of *reorganization*. Such reorganization will itself be part of a broader context of things. To be viable it must not run counter to current macrosocioeconomic structural trends in society. Instead, to a substantial degree reorganization must draw on the same forces for support that are currently contributing to the problem. This is so because these forces are not likely to change soon, and any change in the medical institution—if that change is to be viable—must find support in other aspects of the social structure, just as any other feature of society is so supported. That is to say, rather than attempting to change the structural context in which the problem exists, the view here is that reorganization must take place within that context.

In presenting such a plan I have tried to keep in mind the need for professional autonomy; to place medical professionals in bureaucratic and administrative straitjackets is not likely to lead to the best of medical results. Legislation requiring mandatory service runs counter to basic American values and depending on its form, possibly infringes on constitutional rights. In exchange for such autonomy the medical profession must be willing to assume the responsibility for meeting the needs of society that many members of society believe should be met, and that some are *demanding* with increasing frequency. This will require a degree of reorganization, at least on the part of some members of the medical profession, and in consequence of that, greater organizational constraints on their behavior can be expected. This, in my opinion, is a small price for the medical profession to pay in return for the high degree of autonomy it will still possess. For unless this price is paid, greater constraints on physician behavior may be expected in the future.

Appendix A: Relationships Between Ratio Variables That Have a Common Term

A number of relationships in the study involve ratio variables that have common denominators, such as the relationship between percent urban residents and the physician ratio and between the hospital-bed and physician ratios. Questions about these kinds of correlations were first raised by Karl Pearson (1897), who noted that such correlations may be "spurious," that is, their magnitudes may be artifactually inflated because of the common term. Put somewhat differently, variation in one is to some extent mathematically determined by variation in the other ratio because of the presence of a common term in both.

More recently, economists and sociologists have called attention to the problem. Edwin Kuh and John R. Meyer (1955) note that the statistical analysis of such ratio variables may yield ambiguous results, as do Karl Schuessler (1973) and Glenn V. Fuguitt and Stanley Lieberson (1974). A central issue in all of these works is the conceptual status of ratios, that is, whether it is the ratios or their component parts (numerator and denominator separately) that the investigator is interested in. Consequently, the investigator should state in advance whether the hypothesis to be tested pertains to ratio variables or their component parts. For example, if one is interested in the relationship between national energy consumption and national standard of living, he will usually be interested in the correlation between national per capita energy consumption and per capita gross national product than the correlation between the absolute levels of energy consumption and gross national product. Analysis would be based on ratio (per capita) measures accordingly. The correlation between two ratios (X/Z and Y/Z) may be quite different from the correlation between the numerators of the ratios (X and Y), as can be seen from the following example: Among nations of the world, Kuwait, which has a small population, would rank high on per capita income and energy consumption but low on total national income and energy consumption, whereas the reverse situation would be the case for India, a nation with a large population. In this case, the correlation between ratios would be far more meaningful than the correlation between the numerators.

Or take the crime rate by communities in the United States. It is not the total amount of crime that criminologists are interested in, but the number of crimes (or the number of criminals) as a proportion of the total population. Classifications of different types of crimes for the purpose of developing a causal theory of crime (or theories for different types of crime) may depend on the extent to which different crime rates are intercorrelated (Gibbs 1960). Also, to know the relationship between crimes in a community and the surveillance

227

capacity of the community control system we might want to know the relationship between the number of crimes and, say, the number of police as proportions
of the total population rather than the total number of crimes and total number
of police. In addition, even discounting changes in recording procedures (that
have probably resulted in an increase in the crime rate based on official statistics),
knowledge of changes over time in the total number of crimes committed has
little information value unless it is expressed as a ratio to the total population:
The number of crimes may have increased over time along with the total population, but unless crime figures are expressed as a rate (or as a ratio, percent or
proportion),[a] statements about increases or decreases in crime are difficult to
interpret. And in many instances it is the correlation between the crime rate and
some other ratio variable (percent urban residents) which has total population as
its denominator that is the central interest. Indeed, many of the characteristics
of communities and societies that sociologists are interested in studying—community wealth (per capita income), political participation (e.g., percent of a community who vote), the amount of money a community or society spends for
education, organizational participation (proportion of a community who belong
to one or more formal organizations), unemployment, and the racial, ethnic,
and occupational composition of a population—are ratio variables in which the
total population is usually the denominator, and the theoretically interesting
correlated variables are frequently variables which also have the total population
as the denominator. This is especially true when interest is in the relationship
between various community characteristics and various forms of social pathology,
such as the relationships between population density (number of persons in a
population per square mile, per dwelling, per room) and rates for mortality,
public assistance, juvenile delinquency, and mental hospitalization, all of which
have total population as the denominator or a term that is probably highly correlated with total population (cf. Galle, Gove, and McPherson 1972). The same
is true for the study of other pathologies, such as the relationship between community unemployment and per capita income.

A similar situation exists for physician manpower. It is not the total number
of physicians that is the significant phenomenon but the number of physicians as
a ratio, rate, or proportion of the total population. If the number of physicians
in the United States in 1970 were the same as the number in 1930, the figure
would have a different meaning for the two periods since the same number of
physicians served about 123 million persons in 1930 in comparison to approximately 203 million in 1970. Since the total population of societies and communities vary widely, the total number of physicians is also likely to vary widely,

---

[a]I make no distinction between ratios, rates, proportions, and percents since each is
a function of the relationship between a numerator and a denominator. In this particular
case, the number of physicians in a community can be divided by the total community
population to get a ratio or a proportion, which can be multiplied by a figure 100,000 (or
some other number) to get a rate or by 100 to get a percent.

and a close statistical relationship is apt to exist between them. For example, there are more physicians in Cook County, Illinois than in Davidson County, Tennessee: 10,725 versus 1,170 in Davidson County (Roback 1972, pp. 196-97, 286-87). But in terms of rates (number per 100,000) the supply of physicians is higher in Davidson County: 258 to 194. Or a more obvious example. There are more physicians in India than in Davidson County, but physicians in Davidson County no doubt reach a much higher proportion of their population than do the physicians of India. Therefore, it is the physician ratio that is inherently interesting rather than the absolute number of physicians. For this reason, much of our analysis is based on ratio variables, for physicians as well as other variables. Of course, much of the analysis in this book does not involve correlations between ratios with a common denominator, since a major portion of our analysis includes our index of county wealth, which is measured by median family income. In these instances questions about correlations among ratio variables with common terms do not exist.

Appendix B: Use of Product-Moment and Regression Coefficients

Product-moment and regression coefficients are used in a number of places in this book. Since their use involves several assumptions about the data on which analysis is conducted, a discussion of these assumptions in connection with the data is in order.

One assumption is that measurement is at least at the interval scale level. In all instances where correlation and regression analysis is used in this book, there is no problem in meeting this assumption. Most variables are ratios, proportions, or rates, which are always interval, and of course median family income of counties is an interval measure.

Other assumptions are distribution assumptions. First is the assumption that the form of the regression equation is linear, or the scattergram for the two correlated variables exhibits a linear rather than curvilinear form. Second, the distributions of the independent and dependent variables are normal or bell-shaped, and the joint distribution of the two variables is a bivariate normal distribution. And third, the variances of the dependent distribution is the same for each value of the independent variable, which in technical language is known as homoscedasticity. Whenever the second and third assumptions are met, the first always is, but the reverse is not the case: A linear relationship may occur without the distributions conforming to bivariate normality or homoscedasticity.

Only when analysis is based on a sample of units from a population is it necessary to make all three distribution assumptions. When results are for a probability sample, statistical tests of significiance are usually used, and these are based on a normal (bell-shaped) sampling distribution, which assumes bivariate normality and homoscedasticity. In this way, inferences or generalizations can be made to the population from the sample results with a known probability of error. However, when interest is merely descriptive (rather than inferential), tests of significance are not necessary. This is the case when the entire population rather than a probability sample is the object of investigation. When all units of a population are included in the analysis, results are descriptive of the population and no probability inference is necessary. The regression coefficient describes the best fitting straight line for all the units in the population (e.g., county physician ratio on county median family income), while the product-moment correlation coefficient indicates how closely the units, scatter plotted by the independent and dependent variable values (i.e., counties scatter plotted by community income and physician ratio), deviate from the regression line. Hence, to the extent that the relationship is not linear, the correlation coefficient underestimates the degree of relationship between the two variables. Since in many instances in this book, regression analysis is based on data for entire populations (either of the United States or some particular region or state), use of regression and correlation coefficients in these cases is descriptive, and tests of significance are not usually reported. It is not necessary to assume bivariate normality and homoscedasticity.

However, it is necessary to know how closely bivariate distributions conform to the linear assumption. For unless the relationship is linear, the product-moment correlation coefficient, as a measure of the ability to predict values of the dependent variable from values of the independent variable, is lower than a correlation coefficient that is not restricted by the linear model. Therefore, it is important to know to what extent the correlated variables are linearly related even if analysis is based on an entire population rather than a random or representative sample from the population. For this reason, the product-moment correlation coefficients and correlation ratio are reported. It will be noted, however, that the urban variable, the physician ratio, and hospital-bed ratios are highly skewed, although the distribution of the income variable approximates a bell-shaped (or normal distribution) quite closely (the mean for income is $4,188, with a standard deviation of $1,311; skewness value is 0.176, with 0.0 indicating a perfectly normal distribution.) In spite of the departures from normality of two of the distributions, the scatterdiagrams indicates that the relationships are indeed linear, as is indicated by the fact that the product-moment correlation coefficients and correlation ratios are so similar.

Appendix C: Supplementary Tables

Table C-1
Relationship Between Proportion of County Residents Living in Urban Areas in Physician's County of Origin and County of Practice, in Percentages—Class of 1960

Percent of Residents Living in Urban Areas—County of Practice	Percent of Residents Living in Urban Areas—County of Origin										Total %
	Less Than 10.0	10.0-19.9	20.0-29.9	30.0-39.9	40.0-49.9	50.0-59.9	60.0-69.9	70.0-79.9	80.0-89.9	90 and Above	
90 and above	29.5	18.5	25.3	33.9	30.1	28.7	31.2	32.3	35.6	58.8	44.2
80.0-89.9	20.5	14.8	23.0	18.3	21.6	26.7	14.0	17.7	35.3	17.7	20.9
70.0-79.9	9.0	22.2	6.9	11.0	7.8	8.9	10.8	25.0	7.2	9.8	10.7
60.0-69.9	6.4	7.4	9.2	6.4	11.1	5.9	19.7	8.3	8.1	4.3	7.1
50.0-59.9	9.0	7.4	8.0	6.3	4.6	18.8	6.4	5.7	4.4	2.9	5.1
40.0-49.9	10.3	3.7	12.6	5.5	15.7	4.0	8.3	4.7	5.0	3.3	5.6
30.0-39.9	7.7	11.1	2.3	8.3	4.6	2.0	3.2	3.1	0.9	1.9	2.8
20.0-29.9	3.8	7.4	9.2	3.7	2.6	0.0	3.8	1.0	1.6	0.7	1.8
10.0-19.9	0.0	3.7	2.3	3.7	0.7	3.0	1.3	0.5	0.9	0.2	0.8
10.0 and less	3.8	3.7	1.1	0.9	1.3	2.0	1.3	1.6	0.9	0.5	1.0
D^{a}	0.9235	0.9574	0.9311	0.9064	0.9027	0.8848	0.9098	0.8758	0.8133	0.6768	
N	78	27	87	109	153	101	157	192	320	1,057	

Sources: AAMC Longitudinal Study and U.S. Bureau of the Census (1967).

Note: Percent urban residents for both county of origin and county of practice is for 1960.

[a] D adjusted for maximum value.

Table C-2
Percentage of Physicians Practicing in Communities of Different Sizes Who Came From Cities of Similar Size—Class of 1960

Community Size of Community of Origin	Community Size of Community of Practice										
	Less Than 1,000	1,000-4,999	5,000-9,999	10,000-24,999	25,000-49,999	50,000-99,999	100,000-249,999	250,000-499,999	500,000-999,999	1,000,000 and Above	Total
1,000,000 and above	22.2	18.3	19.7	21.0	16.7	21.3	18.1	14.1	15.6	52.9	20.9
500,000-999,999	11.1	11.1	10.9	9.9	10.3	14.3	10.1	11.3	32.1	11.2	14.3
250,000-499,999	13.9	5.2	8.8	4.6	9.0	4.4	5.9	24.9	7.5	8.2	8.5
100,000-249,999	5.6	7.2	10.2	10.8	10.3	8.8	21.0	12.7	9.6	5.9	10.9
50,000-99,999	22.2	7.2	9.5	8.6	9.3	19.9	8.8	6.1	9.3	5.3	9.9
25,000-49,999	2.8	7.8	4.4	9.9	12.5	7.7	8.4	6.1	5.1	4.1	7.7
10,000-24,999	8.3	14.4	7.3	13.0	9.0	8.1	8.8	10.8	4.8	4.7	8.9
5,000-9,999	0.0	6.5	12.4	8.0	6.1	5.9	5.5	4.7	6.6	2.9	6.3
1,000-4,999	11.1	16.3	13.1	9.0	11.3	6.3	9.7	7.0	7.2	3.5	9.0
Less than 1,000	2.8	5.9	3.6	5.2	5.5	3.3	3.8	2.3	2.1	1.2	3.7
N	35	153	137	324	311	272	238	213	333	170	

Sources: AAMC Longitudinal Study and Rand McNally (1963).

Note: Size of community of practice and size of community of origin are both for 1960.

Table C-3
Regression (b) and Correlation (r) Coefficients Between Residents Living in Urban Areas and Physician Ratios for Six Types of Physicians, 1970-48 Contiguous States

	Regression Coefficient	Correlation Coefficient
Limited specialists	0.738	0.71
Pediatricians	0.110	0.60
Obstetrician-gynecologists	0.113	0.68
Internists	0.251	0.54
General surgeons	0.088	0.45
General practitioners	−0.075	−0.22

Sources: G.A. Roback (1972) and U.S. Bureau of the Census (1972a).

Table C-4
Ratio of Percentage of Physicians Who Originated from Counties of Designated Income Levels to Total 1950 Population, by Median Family Income of Physicians' Counties of Origin—Class of 1960

	Median Income of County of Origin (1969)					
	Less Than $4,000 (16.6)[a]	$4,000-$4,999 (15.8)	$5,000-$5,999 (29.1)	$6,000-$6,999 (24.5)	$7,000 and Above (14.0)	N
Limited specialists	0.51 (8.5)[b]	0.77 (12.1)	1.08 (31.5)	1.39 (34.1)	0.99 (13.8)	1,315
General specialists	0.64 (10.6)	0.80 (12.7)	1.19 (34.5)	1.22 (30.0)	0.89 (12.4)	724
Generalists	1.29 (21.4)	0.96 (15.1)	0.84 (24.5)	1.30 (31.8)	0.51 (7.2)	318

Source: AAMC Longitudinal Study and U.S. Bureau of the Census (1952, 1953; 1967).

[a]Figure in parentheses is percentage of 1950 population living in counties in the column.

[b]Figure in parentheses is percentage of physicians from class of 1960 who originated from counties in the column.

Table C-5

Ratio of Percentage of Physicians Who Originated from Counties of Designated Urban Levels to Total 1950 Population of Counties—Class of 1960

	Percentage of Urban Residents (1967)					
	Less Than 40.0% (21.0)[a]	*40.0%- 59.9% (15.5)*	*60.0%- 79.9% (16.5)*	*80.0%- 89.9% (14.0)*	*90.0%- 100.0% (33.0)*	*N*
Limited specialists	0.54 (11.3)	0.65 (10.1)	0.90 (14.9)	1.06 (14.8)	1.48 (48.7)	1,318
General specialists	0.58 (12.2)	0.70 (10.8)	0.84 (13.8)	0.99 (13.8)	1.50 (49.4)	724
Generalists	1.10 (23.2)	0.95 (14.8)	1.20 (19.8)	0.79 (11.0)	0.94 (31.1)	318

Source: AAMC Longitudinal Study and U.S. Bureau of the Census (1952, 1953; 1967).

[a]Figure in parentheses is percentage of 1950 population living in counties in the column.

[b]Figure in parentheses is percentage of physicians from class of 1960 who originated from counties in the column.

Table C-6

Recruitment-Production Ratios for General and Family Practitioners by Income and Urban Level of Counties—Class of 1960

	Percent Urban Residents (1960)		
Median Annual Family Income (1959)	*Less Than 70.0%*	*70.0-89.9%*	*90.0-100.0%*
$6,000 and above	1.63 (7.99:4.89)[a]	1.07 (16.92:14.29)	0.69 (17.23:24.94)
Less than $6,000	1.19 (40.30:34.58)	0.88 (10.15:11.33)	0.80 (7.38:9.20)

Sources: AAMC Longitudinal Study and U.S. Bureau of the Census (1952, 1953; 1967; 1973a).

[a]Figures in parentheses are percentages of physicians recruited to physicians produced.

Table C-7
Recruitment-Production Ratios for General Specialists by Income and Urban Level of Counties—Class of 1960

Median Annual Family Income (1959)	Percent of Urban Residents (1960)		
	Less Than 70.0%	*70.0-89.9%*	*90.0-100.0%*
$6,000 and above	1.23 (6.01:4.89)[a]	1.26 (19.92:15.75)	1.25 (31.24:24.94)
Less than $6,000	0.53 (18.29:34.58)	0.91 (10.36:11.33)	1.74 (14.91:8.56)

Sources: AAMC Longitudinal Study and U.S. Bureau of the Census (1952, 1953; 1967; 1973a).

[a]Figures in parentheses are percentages of physicians recruited to physicians produced.

Table C-8
Recruitment-Production Ratios for Limited Specialists by Income and Urban Level of Counties—Class of 1960

Median Annual Family Income (1959)	Percent of Urban Residents (1960)		
	Less Than 70.0%[a]	*70.0-89.9%*	*90.0-100.0%*
$6,000 and above	0.96 (4.72:4.89)	1.40 (22.07:15.75)	1.32 (32.56:24.94)
Less than 6,000	0.38 (13.10:24.58)	0.98 (11.14:11.33)	0.90 (16.32:8.56)

Sources: AAMC Longitudinal Study and U.S. Bureau of the Census (1952, 1953; 1967; 1973a).

[a]Figures in parentheses are percentages of physicians recruited to physicians produced.

Table C-9

Percentage of Physicians, by Percentage of Urban Residents in County of Origin, Who Practice in Counties with the Same Level of Urban Residents, by Specialization—Class of 1960

Percent of Urban Residents	Generalists	General Specialists	Limited Specialists	Physicians[a]
90.0%–100.0%	41.8	60.2	60.6	58.8
80.0%–89.9%	40.0	37.1	33.5	35.3
70.0%–79.9%	36.4	34.0	16.7	25.0
60.0%–69.9%	28.6	27.1	12.3	19.7
50.0%–59.9%	36.8	16.0	14.0	18.8
Less than 50.0%	49.4	25.0	14.2	25.1

Sources: AAMC Longitudinal Study and U.S. Bureau of the Census (1967).

[a]From Table C-1.

Table C-10

Relationship Between Specialization and Urban Level of County of Practice for Physicians Who Planned General Practice Careers in 1960—Class of 1960

	Percent Urban Residents (1960)				
	Less Than 50.0%	50.0-69.9%	70.0-79.9%	80.0-89.9%	90.0-100.0%
Speciality[a]	32.6	50.7	56.4	65.8	68.2
Generalist	67.4	49.3	43.4	34.2	31.8
N	135	75	53	79	110

Gamma = 0.32 (x^2 = 44; 3 df; $p < .0001$)

Sources: AAMC Longitudinal Study and U.S. Bureau of the Census (1967).

[a]Includes general and limited specialists.

Bibliography

Alfano, Genrose

    1970   "Nursing in the Decade Ahead," *American Journal of Nursing* 70 (October):2116-18.

American Hospital Association

    1950   "Guide Issue," *Journal of American Hospital Association* 24 (August 1).

    1967   "Guide Issue," *Journal of American Hospital Association* 41 (August 1).

    1969   "Guide Issue," *Journal of American Hospital Association* (August 1).

    1970   "Guide Issue," *Journal of American Hospital Association* (August 1).

American Medical Association

    1959   "Education Issue," *Journal of American Medical Association* (November).

    1960   "Education Issue," *Journal of American Medical Association* (November).

    1961   "Education Issue," *Journal of American Medical Association* (November).

    1962   "Education Issue," *Journal of American Medical Association* (November).

    1963   "Education Issue," *Journal of American Medical Association* (November).

    1964   "Education Issue," *Journal of American Medical Association* (November).

    1965   "Education Issue," *Journal of American Medical Association* (November).

    1966   "Education Issue," *Journal of American Medical Association* (November).

    1967a   "Education Issue," *Journal of American Medical Association* (November).

    1967b   "M.D.'s Obtained for Rural Areas," *The A.M.A. News* (February).

    1968   "Education Issue," *Journal of American Medical Association* (November).

    1971   "Education Issue," *Journal of American Medical Association* (November).

1972 "Education Issue," *Journal of American Medical Association* (November).

1973 "Toward an Explanation of the Geographical Location of Physicians in the United States," in *Contributions to a Comprehensive Health Manpower Strategy.* Chicago: Center for Health Services Research and Development (January):29-67.

American Nurses' Association Special Committee on Allied Nursing Personnel

1966 "Health Occupations Supportive to Nursing," *American Journal of Nursing* 66 (March):559-63.

Anderson, James G., and Harvey H. Marshall

1974 "The Structural Approach to Physician Distribution: A Critical Evaluation," *Health Services Research* 9 (Fall):195-207.

Anderson, Theodore, and Seymour Warkov

1961 "Organizational Size and Functional Complexity: A Study of Administration in Hospitals," *American Sociological Review* 26 (February):23-28.

Bacon, Lloyd

1973 "Migration, Poverty, and the Rural South," *Social Forces* 51 (March):348-55.

Badgley, Robin F., and Samuel Wolfe

1967 *Doctors' Strike.* Toronto: Macmillan Publishers, Inc.

Banfield, Edward

1970 *The Unheavenly City.* Boston: Little, Brown and Company.

Bell, Daniel

1962 *The End of Ideology: On the Exhaustion of Political Ideas in the Fifties.* New York: The Free Press.

Benham, Lee; Alex Maurizi; and Melvin W. Reder

1968 "Migration, Location, and Renumeration of Medical Personnel: Physicians and Dentists," *Review of Economics and Statistics* 50 (August):322-47.

Bice, Thomas W.

1971 *Medical Care for the Disadvantaged: A Survey of Use of Medical Services in Baltimore SMSA.* Baltimore: The Johns Hopkins University Press.

Bible, Bond

1970 "Physicians' Views of Medical Practice in Nonmetropolitan Communities," *Public Health Reports* 81 (January):11-17.

Blalock, Hubert M., Jr.

1965 "Theory Building and the Statistical Concept of Interaction," *American Sociological Review* 30 (June):374-80.

1972 *Social Statistics*, 2nd ed. New York: McGraw-Hill Book Company.

Blau, Peter M.

1960 "Structural Effects," *American Sociological Review* 25 (February):178-93.

1970   "A Formal Theory of Differentiation in Organizations," *American Sociological Review* 35 (April):201-18.

1972   "Interdependence and Hierarchy in Organizations," *Social Science Research* 1 (April):1-24.

Blau, Peter M., and Otis Dudley Duncan

1966   *The American Occupational Structure.* New York: John Wiley & Sons, Inc.

Blau, Peter M., and Richard Schoenherr

1971   *The Structure of Organizations.* New York: Basic Books.

Blumer, Herbert G.

1955   "Attitudes and the Social Act," *Social Problems* 3 (October): 59-65.

Bogue, Donald J.

1969   *Principles of Demography.* New York: John Wiley & Sons.

Bohrnstedt, George W.

1969   "Observations on the Measurement of Change," in Edgar F. Borgatta (ed.), *Sociological Methodology.* San Francisco: Jossey-Bass, Inc., Publishers.

Breisch, W.F.

1970   "Impact of Medical School Characteristics on Location of Physician Practice," *Journal of Medical Education* 45:1068-70.

Brodt, Dagmag E.

1968   "Where is the General Duty Nurse?" *American Journal of Nursing* 68 (August):1732.

Brown, David L.

1972   "The Redistribution of Professional Medical Personnel in Non-metropolitan Wisconsin, 1950-1970." Working Paper, Center for Demography and Ecology. Madison: University of Wisconsin Center for Demography and Ecology.

Carlson, Clifford L., and Gary T. Athelstan

1970   "The Physician's Assistant: Versions and Diversions of a Promising Concept," *Journal of American Medical Association* (December 7): 1855.

Carnegie Commission on Higher Education

1970   *Higher Education and the Nation's Health: Policies for Medical and Dental Education.* New York: McGraw-Hill Book Company.

Carter, Grace M.; David S.C. Chu; John E. Koehler; Robert L. Slighton; and Albert P. Williams, Jr.

1974   *Federal Manpower Legislation and the Academic Health Centers: An Interim Report.* Santa Monica: The Rand Corporation.

Caudill, Harry M.

1973   "O, Appalachia!," *Intellectual Digest* (April):16-19.

Champion, Dean J., and D.B. Olsen

1971   "Physician Behavior in Southern Appalachia: Some Recruitment

Factors," *Journal of Health and Social Behavior* 12 (September): 245-52.

Christman, Luther
    1967   "The role of Systems Engineering in Meeting the Nursing Challenge." Paper presented at the Massachusetts Hospital Association Conference, November 21, Boston, Massachusetts.

Christman, Luther, and Richard C. Jelinek
    1967   "Old Patterns Waste Half the Nursing Hours," *Modern Hospital* 108:78-81.

Coker, R.E.; Norman Miller; Kurt W. Back; and Thomas Donnelly
    1970   "The Medical Student Specialization and General Practice," *North Carolina Medical Journal* 21 (March):96-101.

Coleman, James S.
    1959   *Community Conflict.* Glencoe, Ill.: The Free Press.

Cooper, Barbara, and Nancy Worthington
    1973   "National Health Expenditures, 1919-72," *Social Security Bulletin* (January):3-40.

Cooper, James K.; Karen Heald; and Michael Samuels
    1972   "The Decision for Rural Practice," *Journal of Medical Education* 47 (December):939-44.

Costner, Herbert L.
    1965   "Criteria for Measures of Association," *American Sociological Review* 30 (June):341-53.

Crawford, Rondla L., and Regina C. McCormack
    1971   "Reasons Physicians Leave Primary Practice," *Journal of Medical Education* 46 (April):263-68.

D'Costa, Ayres G., and Rosemary Yancik
    1974   *Association of American Medical Colleges: The Longitudinal Study of Medical School Students of the Class of 1960—Status Report* (May). Washington: American Association of Medical Colleges.

Division of Regional Medical Program
    1969   *Progress Report.* Washington, D.C.: Division of Regional Medical Program.

Duncan, Otis Dudley; Richard Scott; Stanley Lieberson; Beverly Duncan; and Hal H. Winsborough
    1960   *Metropolis and Region.* Baltimore: The Johns Hopkins Press.

Durkheim, Emile
    1937   *The Rules of the Sociological Method.* Chicago: University of Chicago Press.

Ehrenreich, Barbara, and John Ehrenreich
    1970   "Regional Medical Programs: Medical Schools on the Make," in

Barbara Ehrenreich and John Ehrenreich, *The American Health Empire: Power, Profits and Politics*. New York: Random House: 214-31.

Fahs, I.J., and O.L. Peterson
1968   "Towns without Physicians and Towns with Only One—A Study of Four States in the Upper Midwest, 1965," *American Journal of Public Health* 58 (July):1200-1211

Fein, Rashi
1967   *The Doctor Shortage: An Economic Diagnosis*. Washington, D.C.: Brookings Institution.

Fein, Rashi, and Gerald I. Weber
1971   *Financing Medical Education: An Analysis of Alternative Policies and Mechanisms*. A General Report Prepared for the Carnegie Commission on Higher Education and the Commonwealth Fund. New York: McGraw-Hill-Book Company.

Field, Mark G.
1970   "The Medical System and Industrial Society," pp. 143-81 in Alan Sheldon, Frank Baker, and Curtis P. McLaughlin (eds.), *Systems and Medical Care*. Cambridge: The M.I.T. Press.

Fleiss, Joseph L., and Judith M. Tanur
1971   "A Note on the Partial Correlation Coefficient," *The American Statistician* 25 (February):43-45.

Freeman, John H.
1973   "Environment, Technology and the Administrative Intensity of Manufacturing Organizations," *American Sociological Review* 38 (December):750-63.

Freeman, John Henry, and Jerrold E. Dronenfeld
1973   "Problems of Definitional Dependency: The Case of Administrative Intensity," *Social Forces* 52 (September):108-21.

Friedman, Judith J.
1973   "Structural Constraints on Community Action: The Case of Infant Mortality Rates," *Social Problems* 21 (Fall):230-45.

Friedson, Eliot
1960   "Client Control and Medical Practice," *American Journal of Sociology* 65 (January):374-82.
1963   "The Organization of Medical Practice," in Howard E. Freeman, Sol Levine, and Leo G. Reeder (eds.), *Handbook of Medical Sociology*. Englewood Cliffs, N.J.: Prentice-Hall.

Fuguitt, Glenn V., and Stanley Lieberson
1974   "Correlations of Ratios or Difference Scores having Common Terms," in Herbert L. Costner (ed.), *Sociological Methodology, 1973-74*. San Francisco: Jossey-Bass, Inc.

Galle, Omer R.; Walter R. Gove; and Miller J. McPherson
    1972   "Population Density and Pathology: What are the Relationships
            for Man?" *Science* 176 (April):23-30.

Gibbs, Jack P.
    1960   "Needed: Analytical Typologies in Criminology," *Southwestern
            Social Science Quarterly* 40 (March):321-29.

Gibbs, Jack P., and Walter T. Martin
    1960   "Urbanization, Technology, and the Division of Labor," *American
            Sociological Review* 27 (October):667-77.

Ginzburg, Eli, and Miriam Ostow
    1969   *Men, Money and Medicine.* New York: Columbia University Press.

Greenhill, Stanley, and Harry J. Singh
    1964   "Comparison of the Function of Medical Practitioners in Rural
            Areas with Those in Urban Areas," *Journal of Medical Education*
            39:806-9.
    1965   "Comparison of the Professional Functions of Rural and Urban
            General Practitioners," *Journal of Medical Education* 40 (Septem-
            ber):856-61.

Haas, Eugene R.; Richard H. Hall; and N.J. Johnson
    1963   "The Size of the Supportive Component in Organizations: A
            Multi-organizational Analysis," *Social Forces* 42 (October):9-17.

Hall, Oswald
    1946   "The Informal Organization of the Medical Profession," *Canadian
            Journal of Economics and Political Science* 12 (February):30-41.
    1948   "The Stages of a Medical Career," *American Journal of Sociology*
            53 (March):327-36.

Hamilton, C. Horace
    1965   "Educational Selectivity of Migration from Farm to Urban to
            Other Nonfarm Communities," in Mildred B. Kantor (ed.),
            Mobility and Mental Health. Springfield, Illinois: Charles C.
            Thomas.

Hansen, Niles M.
    1970   *Rural Poverty and the Urban Crisis: A Strategy for Regional
            Development.* Bloomington: Indiana University Press.

Hassinger, Edward L.
    1963   *Socio-Economic Backgrounds and Community Orientation of
            Rural Physicians.* University of Missouri Agricultural Experiment
            Station Research Bulletin 822. Columbia: University of Missouri
            Press.

Haug, J.N.; G.A. Roback; and B.C. Martin
    1971   *Distribution of Physicians in the United States, 1970.* Chicago:
            American Medical Association.

Haug, J.N.; G.A. Roback; C.N. Theodore; and B.E. Balfe
    1970   *Distribution of Physicians, Hospitals and Hospital Beds in the U.S.:*

Regional, State, County, Metropolitan Areas. Chicago: American Medical Association.

1971   *Distribution of Physicians, Hospitals, and Hospital Beds in the U.S., 1968.* Chicago: American Medical Association.

Hawley, Amos; William Boland; and Margaret Boland

1965   "Population Size and Administration in Institutions of Higher Education," *American Sociological Review* 30 (April):252-55.

Health Services and Mental Health Administration

1972   *Hill-Burton Project Register, July 1, 1964-June 30, 1971.*

Held, Philip J.

1973   *The Migration of the 1955-1965 Graduates of American Medical Schools.* Berkeley: Ford Foundation Program Research in University Administration.

Heydebrand, Wolf

1973   *Hospital Bureaucracy: A Comparative Study of Organizations* New York: Dunellen Publishing Company.

Hoselitz, Bert F.

1967   *A Reader's Guide to the Social Sciences.* New York: The Free Press.

Hunter, Floyd

1953   *Community Power Structure: A Study of Decision Makers.* Chapel Hill: University of North Carolina Press.

Hyman, Herbert

1955   *Survey Design and Analysis: Principles, Cases and Procedures.* Glencoe, Ill.: The Free Press.

Jacoby, Neil H.

1973   *Corporate Power and Social Responsibility: A Blueprint for the Future.* New York: Macmillan Publishers, Inc.

Joroff, Sheila, and Vicente Navorro

1971   "Medical Manpower: A Multivariate Analysis of the Distribution of Physicians in Urban United States," *Medical Care* 9 (September-October):428-38.

Kaplan, Roy H.

1970   "Health Care in America: Anarchonistic and Inequitable." Paper read at the 65th annual meeting of the American Sociological Association, Washington, D.C. (September).

Kaufman, Harold F.

1959   "Toward an Interactional Conception of Community," *Social Forces* 38 (October):8-17.

Kessel, Reuben A.

1970   "The AMA and the Supply of Physicians," *Law and Contemporary Problems* 35 (Spring):267-83.

Klatzky, S.R.

1970   "Organizational Inequality: The Case of the Public Employment

Agencies," *American Journal of Sociology* 76 (November): 474-91.

Krause, Eliot A.
    1971   *The Sociology of Occupations.* Boston: Little, Brown and Company.

Kuh, Edwin, and John R. Meyer
    1955   "Correlation and Regression Estimates when the Data are Ratios," *Econometrica* 23 (March):400-416.

Last, J.M.
    1967   "Regional Distribution of General Practitioners and Consultants in the National Health Service," *British Medical Journal* 2 (June 24):796-99.

Lerner, Monroe, and Odin Anderson
    1963   *Health Progress in the United States: 1900-1960.* Chicago: Health Information Foundation.

Levine, H.G.
    1970   "In Review: The Manpower Shortage," *The American Journal of Medical Technology* 36 (May):254-63.

Lysault, Jerome P.
    1970   *An Abstract for Action.* New York: McGraw-Hill Book Company.

Lyford, Joseph
    1962   *The Talk of Vandalia.* New York: Harper & Row.

MacQueen, John C.
    1968   "A Study of Iowa Medical Physicians," *Journal of Iowa Medical Society* (November):1129-35.

Marden, Parker G.
    1966   "A Demographic and Ecological Analysis of the Distribution of Physicians in Metropolitan America, 1960," *American Journal of Sociology* 72 (November):290-300.

Marshall, Carter L.; Khatab M. Hassanein; Ruth S. Hassanein; and Carol L. Marshall
    1971   "Principle Components Analysis of the Distribution of Physicians, Dentists, and Osteopaths in a Western State," *American Journal of Public Health* 61 (August):1556-64.

Martin, E.D.; R.E. Moffata; R.T. Falter; and J.D. Walder
    1968   "Where Graduates Go. The University of Kansas School of Medicine: A Study of the Profiles of 959 Graduates and Factors which Influenced the Geographic Distribution," *Journal of Kansas Medical Society* 69 (March):84-89.

Martindale, Don, and R. Galen Hanson
    1969   *Small Town and the Nation: The Conflict of Local and Translocal Forces.* Westport, Connecticut: Greenwood Publishing Corporation.

Mauksch, Hans

 1965 "The Nurse: Coordinator of Patient Care," in James Skipper and Robert Leonard (eds.), *Social Interaction and Patient Care.* Philadelphia, J.B. Lippincott Company:251-66.

Mayhew, Bruce H., and William A. Rushing

 1973 "Occupational Structure of General Hospitals: The Harmonic Series Model," *Social Forces* 52 (September):455-61.

McNamara, Mary E., and Clifford Todd

 1970 "A Survey of Group Practice in the United States, 1969," *American Journal of Public Health* (July):1304.

McNerney, Walter J., and Donald G. Riedel

 1962 *Regionalization and Health Care: An Experiment in Three Communities,* Ann Arbor: The University of Michigan Press.

Medical Economics

 1969 "Does Your State Produce its Share of Physicians?" *Medical Economics* (December):100-01.

Melloan, George

 1973 "Cooling Down Health Care's Crisis Rhetoric," *The Wall Street Journal* (March 1):6.

Merton, Robert K.

 1957 *Social Theory and Social Structure*, rev. ed. Glencoe: The Free Press.

Miles, David L., and William A. Rushing

 1975 "A Study of Physician's Assistants in a Rural Setting" (forthcoming).

Mountin, John W.; Elliott H. Pennell; and G.S. Brockett

 1945 "Location and Movement of Physicians, 1923 and 1938—Changes in Urban and Rural Totals for Established Physicians," *Public Health Reports* 60 (February 16):173-85.

Mountin, Joseph W.; Elliott H. Pennell; and Virginia Nicolay

 1942a "Location and Movement of Physicians 1923 and 1938—Effect of Local Factors on Location," *Public Health Reports* 57 (December 18):1945-53.

 1942b "Location and Movement of Physicians, 1923 and 1938—General Observations," *Public Health Reports* 57 (September 11):1362-75.

 1942c "Location and Movement of Physicians, 1923 and 1938—Turnover as a Factor Affecting State Totals," *Public Health Reports* 57 (November 20):1752-61.

Mueller, John H.; Karl F. Schuessler; and Herbert L. Coster

 1970 *Statistical Reasoning in Sociology.* Boston: Houghton-Mifflin Company.

Nashville Tennessean

 1973 January 24.

National Academy of Sciences – Institute of Medicine
   1974   *Costs of Education in the Health Professions: Report of a Study,*
           Parts I and II. Washington, D.C.: National Academy of Sciences.
National Advisory Commission on Health Manpower
   1967   *Report of the National Advisory Commission on Health Man-*
           power, Vol. I. Washington, D.C.: U.S. Government Printing
           Office.
   1967   *Report of the National Advisory Commission on Health Man-*
           power, Vol. II. Washington, D.C.: U.S. Government Printing
           Office.
Nisbet, Robert N.
   1971   "Introduction," in Robert K. Merton and Robert N. Nisbet,
           Contemporary Social Problems, 3rd. ed. New York: Harcourt
           Brace Jovanovich, Inc.
Office of Comprehensive Health Planning, Tennessee Department of Public
   Health
   1970   *Physicians in Tennessee, 1969.* Nashville: Office of Comprehen-
           sive Health Planning and Tennessee Department of Public Health.
Owens, Arthur
   1970   "General Surgeons: Too Many in the Wrong Places," *Medical*
           Economics (July 20):128-33.
Palmore, Erdman B., and Phillip E. Hammond
   1964   "Interaction Factors in Juvenile Delinquency," *American Socio-*
           logical Review 29 (December):848-54.
Parker, Ralph C.; Richard A. Rix; and Thomas G. Tuxhill
   1969   "Social and Demographic Factors Effecting Physician Location
           in Upstate New York," *New York State Journal of Medicine* 69
           (March):706-12.
Parker, Ralph C. and Thomas G. Tuxhill
   1967   "The Attitudes of Physicians Toward Small Town Community
           Practice," *Journal of Medical Education* 42 (April):327-44.
Paxton, Harry T.
   1969   "Private Group Practice: First Choice for the Future?" *Hospital*
           Physicians (February):60.
Pearson, Karl
   1897   "Mathematical Contribution to the Theory of Evolution–On a
           Form of Spurious Correlation Which May Arise When Indices
           Are Used in the Measurement of Organs," *Proceedings of the*
           Royal Society of London 60:489-98.
Pennell, Maryland Y., and Marion E. Altenderfer
   1952   *Health Manpower Source Book,* Section 1, Physicians. Washing-
           ton, D.C.: U.S. Government Printing Office.

1954   *Health Manpower Source Book,* Section 4, County Data from
            1950 Census and Area Analysis. Wahington, D.C.: U.S. Govern-
            ment Printing Office.

Pennell, Maryland Y., and Kathryn I. Baker
1965   *Health Manpower Source Book,* Section 19, Location of Man-
            power in 8 Health Occupations, 1962. Washington, D.C.: U.S.
            Government Printing Office.

Rand McNally
1963   *Road Atlas for Canada, the United States and Mexico.* Chicago:
            Rand McNally.

Reiss, Albert J., Jr.
1954   "Some Logical and Methodological Problems in Community
            Research." *Social Forces* 33 (October):51-57.

1966   "The Sociological Study of Communities," pp. 591-603 in Roland
            L. Warren (ed.), *Perspectives on the American Community: A
            Book of Readings.* Chicago: Rand McNally.

Reskin, Barbara, and Frederick L. Campbell
1974   "Physician Distribution Across Metropolitan Areas," *American
            Journal of Sociology* 79 (January):981-98.

Rice, Dorothy P. and Barbara S. Cooper
1973   "National Health Expenditures, 1929-72," *Social Security Bul-
            letin* (January):3-40.

Rimlinger, Gaston V., and Henry B. Steele
1963   "An Economic Interpretation of the Spatial Distribution of
            Physicians in the U.S.," *Southern Economic Journal* 30 (July):
            1-12.

Roback, G.A.
1972   *Distribution of Physicians in the U.S., 1971.* Chicago: American
            Medical Association.

Ross, Edward Alsworth
1925   *The Outlines of Sociology.* New York: The Century Co.

Rushing, William A.
1971   "Public Policy, Community Constraints, and the Distribution of
            Medical Resources," *Social Problems* 19 (Summer):21-36.

1973   "Physicians and Size of Community of Practice: Analysis of
            AAMC Data" (unpublished manuscript).

Rushing, William A., and David L. Miles
1975   "Effects of Health Insurance and Health Status on Physician
            Visits." Paper presented at the 1975 meetings of the American
            Public Health Association, Chicago, Illinois.

Rutstein, David D.
1967   *The Coming Revolution in Medicine.* Cambridge: The M.I.T. Press.

Sadler, Alfred M., Jr.; Blair L. Sadler; and Ann A. Bliss
    1972   *The Physician's Assistant: Today and Tomorrow.* New Haven:
              Yale University Press.
Schuessler, Karl
    1973   "Ratio Variables and Path Models," in Arthur S. Goldberger and
              Otis Dudley Duncan (eds.), *Structural Equation Models in the
              Social Sciences.* New York: Seminar Press.
Schwartz, Harry
    1972   *The Care for American Medicine: A Realistic Look at Our Health
              Care System.* New York: David McKay and Company, Inc.
Selznick, Philip
    1949   *TVA and the Grass Roots.* Berkeley: University of California
              Press.
Shortell, Stephen M.
    1973   "Patterns of Referral Among Internists in Private Practice: A
              Social Exchange Model," *Journal of Health and Social Behavior*
              14 (December):335-48.
    1974   "Determinants of Physician Referral Rates: An Exchange Theory
              Approach," *Medical Care* 12 (January):13-31.
Sloan, Frank A.
    1968   *Economic Models of Physician Supply.* Ph.D. dissertation, Depart-
              ment of Economics, Harvard University.
Somers, Ann R.
    1968   "Some Basic Determinants of Medical Care and Health Policy,"
              Millbank Memorial Fund Quarterly 46 (January):13-31.
Somers, Herman Miles, and Ann Ramsey Somers
    1961   *Doctors, Patients and Health Insurance.* Washington, D.C.: Brook-
              ings Institutions.
Star, Jack
    1971   "Where have our Doctors Gone?" *Look* 35 (June 29):15-17.
Steele, Henry B., and Gaston V. Rimlinger
    1965   "Income Opportunities and Physician Location Trends in the
              United States," *Western Economic Journal* (Spring):182-94.
Stephan, G. Edward
    1971   "Variation in County Size: A Theory of Segmental Growth,"
              American Sociological Review 36 (June):451-60.
Stewart, William H., and Maryland Y. Pennell
    1960   *Health Manpower Source Book,* Section 10, Physicians' Age,
              Type of Practice, and Location. Washington, D.C.: U.S. Govern-
              ment Printing Office.
Strickland, Stephen P.
    1972   *U.S. Health Care: What's Wrong and What's Right.* New York:
              Universe Books.

Surgeon General's Consultant Group on Medical Education
    1959   *Physicians for a Growing America*. Washington, D.C.: U.S.
            Government Printing Office.

Tennessee Department of Public Health
    1950   *Annual Report of Hospitals in Tennessee*. Nashville: Tennessee
            Department of Public Health.
    1968   *Annual Report of Hospitals in Tennessee*. Nashville: Tennessee
            Department of Public Health.

Tennessee Higher Education Commission
    1970   "Survey of Medical Education in Tennessee: A Preliminary
            Report" (Nashville).

Terris, Milton, and Mary Monk
    1956   "Recent Trends in the Distribution of Physicians in Upstate
            New York," *American Journal of Public Health* 46 (May).

Theodore, C.N., and J.N. Haug
    1968   *Selected Characteristics of the Physician Population, 1963 and
            1967*. Chicago: American Medical Association.

Theodore, C.N.; G.E. Sutter; and J.N. Haug
    1968   *Medical School Alumni, 1967*. Chicago: American Medical
            Association.

Theodore, C.N., and G.E. Sutter
    1966   *Distribution of Physicians, Hospitals, and Hospital Beds in U.S.
            (1965) by Census Region, State, County and Metropolitan Area*.
            Chicago: American Medical Association.

Theodore, C.N.; G.E. Sutter; and E.A. Jokiel
    1967   *Distribution of Physicians, Hospitals, and Hospital Beds in the
            U.S., 1966, Vol. 1, Regional, State, County*. Chicago: American
            Medical Association.

Thompson, James D.
    1967   *Organizations in Action*, New York: McGraw-Hill Book Company.
    1973   "Society's Frontiers for Organizing Activities," *Public Adminis-
            tration Review* 33 (July/August):327-35.

Thompson, Wilbur R.
    1969   "The Economic Base of Urban Problems," in Neal W. Chamber-
            lain (ed.), *Contemporary Economic Issues*. Homewood Illinois:
            Richard D. Irwin, Inc.

U.S. Bureau of the Census
    1952   *U.S. Census of Population*, Vol. 1. *Characteristics of the Popula-
    1953   tion*, Parts 2-51, excluding Part 3 (Alaska), 10 (District of
            Columbia), 13 (Hawaii), and 48 (Virginia). Washington, D.C.:
            U.S. Government Printing Office.
    1953   *U.S. Census of the Population: 1950*, Vol. 1. *Characteristics of
            the Population*, Part 44, Tennessee.

1962   *U.S. Census of Population,* Vol. 1. *Characteristics of the Popu-*
1963   *lation,* Parts 2-51, excluding Part 3 (Alaska), 10 (District of
              Columbia), 13 (Hawaii), and 48 (Virginia). Washington, D.C.:
              U.S. Government Printing Office.
1963a   *U.S. Census of Population: 1960. Subject Reports. Occupa-*
              tional Characteristics. Final Report PC(2)-7A. Washington, D.C.:
              U.S. Government Printing Office.
1963b   *U.S. Census of Population: 1960,* Vol. 1. *Characteristics of the*
              Population, Part 44. Tennessee. Wahington, D.C.: U.S. Govern-
              ment Printing Office.
1964   *U.S. Census of Population: 1960,* Vol. I. *Characteristics of the*
              Population, Part I. United States Summary. Washington, D.C.:
              U.S. Government Printing Office.
1967   *County and City Data Book, 1967* (A Statistical Abstract Supple-
              ment). Washington, D.C.: U.S. Government Printing Office.
1971   *The American Almanac: The U.S. Book of Facts, Statistics and*
              Information. New York: Grosset and Dunlap.
1971   *U.S. Census of Population: 1970,* Vol. 1. *Characteristics of the*
1972   *Population,* Parts 2-51, excluding Part 3 (Alaska), 10 (District of
              Columbia), 13 (Hawaii), and 48 (Virginia). Washington, D.C.:
              U.S. Government Printing Office.
1972a   *General Population Characteristics: United States Summary,*
              Final Report PC(1) - B1, Washington, D.C.: U.S. Government
              Printing Office.
1972b   *General Social and Economic Characteristics.* United States
              Summary. Washington, D.C.: U.S. Government Printing Office.
1973a   *County and City Data Book, 1972* (A Statistical Abstract Supple-
              ment). Washington, D.C.: U.S. Government Printing Office.
1973b   *Statistical Abstract of the United States: 1973* (94th ed.). Wash-
              ington, D.C.: U.S. Government Printing Office.
U.S. Public Health Service
1965   *Health Resources Statistics.* Washington, D.C.: U.S. Government
              Printing Office.
Warren, Roland L.
1972   *The Community in America,* 2nd ed. Chicago: Rand McNally.
Weiskotten, Herman G.; Walter S. Wiggins; Marion E. Altenderfer; Marjorie Gouch;
  and Ann Tipner
1960   "Trends in Medical Practice—An Analysis of the Distribution of
              Characteristics of Medical College Graduates, 1915-1950," *Journal*
              of Medical Education 35 (December):1071-1121.
West, James
1945   *Plainville, U.S.A.* New York: Columbia University Press.

Williams, R.C., and W.E. Uzzell

    1960   "Attracting Physicians to Smaller Communities," *Hospitals* 34:
              49-51.

Yett, Donald E., and Frank A. Sloan

    1971   "Analysis of Migration Patterns of Recent Medical School
              Graduates." Paper read at the Health Services Research Con-
              ference on Factors in Health Manpower Performance and Delivery
              of Health Care, Department of Health, Education and Welfare,
              National Center for Health Services Research and Development,
              Chicago.

Zentner, Harry

    1973   *Prelude to Administrative Theory: Essays in Social Structure*
              and Social Process. Galgary: Strayer Publications, Limited.

About the Author

William A. Rushing is professor of sociology at Vanderbilt University; he received the Ph.D. from the University of North Carolina in 1961. He is the author of three other books—*The Psychiatric Professions: Power, Conflict, and Adaptation in a Psychiatric Hospital Staff; Deviant Behavior and Social Process;* and *Class, Culture and Alienation.* He is also the author of numerous articles which have appeared in the *American Sociological Review, The American Journal of Sociology, Administrative Science Quarterly, Journal of Health and Social Behavior, Health Services Research* and other journals. He has been consultant to a number of private and public agencies, including the National Institute of Health, National Institute of Mental Health, National Center for Health Services Research, and the National Academy of Sciences. He is a member of the National Academy of Sciences-National Research Council Committee to Study Health Care Resources in the Veterans Administration.